Current Clinical Strategies

Pediatrics

2007 Edition

Paul D. Chan, MD

Current Clinical Strategies Publishing

www.ccspublishing.com/ccs

Digital Book and Updates

Purchasers of this book can download the digital version and updates at the Current Clinical Strategies Publishing web site:

www.ccspublishing.com/ccs/ped.htm.

Current Clinical Strategies Publishing
27071 Cabot Road
Laguna Hills, California 92653
Phone: 800.331.8227
Fax: 800.965.9420
Internet: www.ccspublishing.com/ccs
E-mail: info@ccspublishing.com

Printed in USA

ISBN 1-929622-76-7

Contents

General Pediatrics

Pediatric History and Physical Examination

History

Identifying Data: Patient's name, age, sex. List the patient's significant medical problems. Name and relationship of informant (patient, parent).

Chief Compliant: Reason given for seeking medical care and the duration of the symptom(s).

History of Present Illness (HPI): Describe the course of the patient's illness, including when it began, character of the symptoms; aggravating or alleviating factors; pertinent positives and negatives. Past diagnostic testing.

Past Medical History (PMH): Past diseases, surgeries, hospitalizations; medical problems; history of asthma.

Birth History: Gestational age at birth, preterm, obstetrical problems.

Developmental History: Motor skills, language development, self-care skills.

Medications: Include prescription and OTC drugs, vitamins, herbal products, natural remedies, nutritional supplements.

Feedings: Diet, volume of formula per day.

Immunizations: Up to date?

Drug Allergies: Penicillin, codeine?

Food Allergies:

Family History: Medical problems in family, including the patient's disorder. Asthma, cancer, tuberculosis, allergies.

Social History: Family situation, alcohol, smoking, drugs. Level of education.

Review of Systems (ROS):

    General: Weight loss, fever, chills, fatigue, night sweats.

    Skin: Rashes, skin discolorations.

    Head: Headaches, dizziness, seizures.

    Eyes: Visual changes.

    Ears: Tinnitus, vertigo, hearing loss.

    Nose: Nose bleeds, discharge.

    Mouth and Throat: Dental disease, hoarseness, throat pain.

    Respiratory: Cough, shortness of breath, sputum (color and consistency).

    Cardiovascular: Dyspnea on exertion, edema, valvular disease.

    Gastrointestinal: Abdominal pain, vomiting, diarrhea, constipation.

    Genitourinary: Dysuria, frequency, hematuria.

    Gynecological: Last menstrual period (frequency, duration), age of menarche; dysmenorrhea, contraception, vaginal bleeding.

    Endocrine: Polyuria, polydipsia.

Pediatric History and Physical Examination

Musculoskeletal: Joint pain or swelling, arthritis, myalgias.
Skin and Lymphatics: Easy bruising, lymphadenopathy.
Neuropsychiatric: Weakness, seizures.
Pain: quality (sharp/stabbing, aching, pressure), location, duration

Physical Examination

General appearance: Note whether the patient looks "ill," well, or malnourished.
Physical Measurements: Weight, height, head circumference (plot on growth charts).
Vital Signs: Temperature, heart rate, respiratory rate, blood pressure.
Skin: Rashes, scars, moles, skin turgor, capillary refill (in seconds).
Lymph Nodes: Cervical, axillary, inguinal nodes: size, tenderness.
Head: Bruising, masses, fontanels.
Eyes: Pupils: equal, round, and reactive to light and accommodation (PERRLA); extra ocular movements intact (EOMI). Funduscopy (papilledema, hemorrhages, exudates).
Ears: Acuity, tympanic membranes (dull, shiny, red, intact, bulging, injected).
Mouth and Throat: Mucus membrane color and moisture; oral lesions, dentition, pharynx, tonsils.
Neck: Thyromegaly, lymphadenopathy, masses.
Chest: Equal expansion, rhonchi, crackles, rubs, breath sounds.
Heart: Regular rate and rhythm (RRR), first and second heart sounds (S1, S2); gallops (S3, S4), murmurs (grade 1-6), pulses (graded 0-2+).
Breast: Discharge, masses; axillary masses.
Abdomen: Bowel sounds, bruits, tenderness, masses; hepatomegaly, splenomegaly; guarding, rebound, percussion note (tympanic), suprapubic tenderness.
Genitourinary: Inguinal masses, hernias, scrotum, testicles.
Pelvic Examination: Vaginal mucosa, cervical discharge, uterine size, masses, adnexal masses.
Extremities: Joint swelling, range of motion, edema (grade 1-4+); cyanosis, clubbing, edema (CCE); pulses.
Rectal Examination: Sphincter tone, masses, fissures; test for occult blood
Neurological: Mental status and affect; gait, strength (graded 0-5), sensation, deep tendon reflexes (biceps, triceps, patellar, ankle; graded 0-4+).
Labs: Electrolytes (sodium, potassium, bicarbonate, chloride, BUN, creatinine), CBC (hemoglobin, hematocrit, WBC count, platelets, differential); x-rays, ECG, urine analysis (UA), liver function tests (LFTs).
Assessment (Impression): Assign a number to each problem and discuss separately. Discuss differential diagnosis and give reasons that support the working diagnosis; give reasons for excluding other diagnoses.
Plan: Describe therapeutic plan for each numbered problem, including testing, laboratory studies, medications.

Progress Notes

Daily progress notes should summarize developments in a patient's hospital course, problems that remain active, plans to treat those problems, and arrangements for discharge. Progress notes should address every element of the problem list.

Example Progress Note

Date/time:
Identify Specialty and Level of Education: eg, Pediatric resident PL-3
Subjective: Any problems and symptoms of the patient should be charted. Appetite, pain, or fussiness may be included.
Objective:
General appearance.
Vitals, including highest temperature (T^{max}) over past 24 hours.
Feedings, fluid inputs and outputs (I/O), including oral and parenteral intake and urine and stool volume output.
Physical exam, including chest and abdomen, with particular attention to active problems. Emphasize changes from previous physical exams.
Labs: Include new test results and circle abnormal values.
Current Medications: List all medications and dosages.
Assessment and Plan: A separate assessment and plan should be written for each problem.

Discharge Note

The discharge note should be written in the patient's chart prior to discharge.

Discharge Note

Date/time:
Diagnoses:
Treatment: Briefly describe treatment provided during hospitalization, including surgical procedures and antibiotic therapy.
Studies Performed: Electrocardiograms, CT scans, CXR.
Discharge Medications:
Follow-up Arrangements:

Prescription Writing

- Patient's name:
- Date:
- Drug name, dosage form, dose, route, frequency (include concentration for oral liquids or mg strength for oral solids): Amoxicillin 125mg/5mL 5 mL PO tid
- Quantity to dispense: mL for oral liquids, # of oral solids
- Refills: If appropriate
- Signature

Procedure Note

A procedure note should be written in the chart after a procedure is performed (eg lumbar puncture).

Procedure Note

Date and Time:
Procedure:
Indications:
Patient Consent: Document that the indications, risks and alternatives to the procedure were explained to the parents and patient. Note that the parents and the patient were given the opportunity to ask questions and that the parents consented to the procedure in writing.
Lab tests: Relevant labs, such as the CBC
Anesthesia: Local with 2% lidocaine
Description of Procedure: Briefly describe the procedure, including sterile prep, anesthesia method, patient position, devices used, anatomic location of procedure, and outcome.
Complications and Estimated Blood Loss (EBL):
Disposition: Describe how the patient tolerated the procedure.
Specimens: Describe any specimens obtained and lab tests that were ordered.

Developmental Milestones

Age	Milestones
1 month	Raises head slightly when prone; alerts to sound; regards face, moves extremities equally.
2-3 months	Smiles, holds head up, coos, reaches for familiar objects, recognizes parent.
4-5 months	Rolls front to back and back to front; sits well when propped; laughs, orients to voice; enjoys looking around; grasps rattle, bears some weight on legs.
6 months	Sits unsupported; passes cube hand to hand; babbles; uses raking grasp; feeds self crackers.
8-9 months	Crawls, cruises; pulls to stand; pincer grasp; plays pat-a-cake; feeds self with bottle; sits without support; explores environment.
12 months	Walking, talking a few words; understands "no"; says "mama/dada" discriminately; throws objects; imitates actions, marks with crayon, drinks from a cup.
15-18 months	Comes when called; scribbles; walks backward; uses 4-20 words; builds tower of 2 blocks.
24-30 months	Removes shoes; follows 2 step command; jumps with both feet; holds pencil, knows first and last name; knows pronouns. Parallel play; points to body parts, runs, spoon feeds self, copies parents.
3 years	Dresses and undresses; walks up and down steps; draws a circle; uses 3-4 word sentences; takes turns; shares. Group play.
4 years	Hops, skips, catches ball; memorizes songs; plays cooperatively; knows colors; copies a circle; uses plurals.
5 years	Jumps over objects; prints first name; knows address and mother's name; follows game rules; draws three part man; hops on one foot.

Immunizations

Immunization Schedule for Infants and Children		
Age	**Immunizations**	**Comments**
Birth - 2 months	HBV	If mother is HbsAg positive or unknown status, the first dose of HBV should be given within 12 hours of birth along with hepatitis B immune globulin 0.5 mL.
1-4 months	HBV	The second HBV dose should be given at least one month after the first dose. For infants of HbsAg positive or unknown status mothers, the second dose should be given at 1-2 months of age.
2 months	DTaP, Hib, IPV, PCV	DTP and Hib are available combined as Tetramune.
4 months	DTaP, Hib, IPV, PCV	
6 months	DTaP, (Hib), PCV	Dose 3 of Hib is not indicated if doses 1 and 2 were PedvaxHIB.
6-18 months	HBV, IPV	The third HBV dose should be administered at least 4 months after the first dose and at least 2 months after the second dose. For infants of HbsAg positive or unknown status mothers, the third dose should be given at 6 months of age.
12-15 months 12-18 months	Hib, PCV, MMR VAR	Tuberculin testing may be done at the same visit if indicated. Varicella vaccine is recommended in children who do not have a reliable history of having had the clinical disease.
15-18 months	DTaP	The 4th dose of DTaP should be given 6-12 months after the third dose of DTaP and may be given as early as 12 months, provided that the interval between doses 3 and 4 is at least 6 mo.
4-6 years	DTaP, IPV, MMR	DTaP and IPV should be given at or before school entry. DTaP should not be given after the 7th birthday

Age	Immunizations	Comments
11-12 years	MMR	Omit if MMR dose was given at age 4-6 years.
14-16 years	Td	Repeat every 10 years throughout life

HBV = Hepatitis B virus vaccine; DTaP = diphtheria and tetanus toxoids and acellular pertussis vaccine; Hib = Haemophilus influenzae type b conjugate vaccine; IPV = inactivated polio vaccine; MMR = live measles, mumps, and rubella viruses vaccine; PCV = pneumococcal conjugate vaccine (Prevnar); Td = adult tetanus toxoid (full dose) and diphtheria toxoid (reduced dose), for children >7 year and adults; VAR = varicella virus vaccine

Recommended Schedule for Children Younger than 7 Years Not Immunized in the First Year of Life

Age	Immunizations	Comments
First visit	DTaP, (Hib), HBV, MMR, IPV, (PCV), VAR	If indicated, tuberculin testing may be done at the same visit. If child is ≥5 years, Hib is not indicated. Pneumococcal conjugate vaccine recommended for all children <2 years or 24-59 months of age and at high risk for invasive pneumococcal disease (eg sickle cell anemia, HIV, immunocompromised). Varicella vaccine if child has not had varicella disease.
Interval after 1st visit 1 month 2 months ≥8 months	DTaP, HBV DTaP, Hib, IPV, (PCV) DTaP, HBV, IPV	Second dose of Hib is indicated only if first dose was received when <15 months. Second dose of PCV 6-8 weeks after first dose (if criteria met above).
4-6 years (at or before school entry)	DTaP, IPV, MMR	DTaP is not necessary if the fourth dose was given after the fourth birthday. IPV is not necessary if the third dose was given after the fourth birthday.
11-12 years	MMR	MMR should be given at entry to middle school or junior high school if it wasn't given at age 4-6 years.
10 years later	Td	Repeat every 10 years

HBV = Hepatitis B virus vaccine; DTaP = diphtheria and tetanus toxoids and acellular pertussis vaccine; Hib = Haemophilus influenzae type b conjugate vaccine; IPV = inactivated polio vaccine; MMR = live measles, mumps, and rubella viruses vaccine; PCV = pneumococcal conjugate vaccine (Prevnar); Td = adult tetanus toxoid and diphtheria toxoid; VAR = varicella virus vaccine

Recommended Schedule for Children >7 Years Who Were Not Immunized Previously

Age	Immunizations	Comments
First visit	HBV, IPV, MMR, Td, VAR	Varicella vaccine if child has not had varicella disease.
Interval after First visit 2 months 8-14 months	HBV, IPV, Td, VAR, MMR HBV, Td, IPV	If child is $\geq$13 years old, a second varicella vaccine dose is needed 4-8 weeks after the first dose.
11-12 years old	MMR	Omit if MMR dose was given at age 4-6 years.
10 years later	Td	Repeat every 10 years

HBV = Hepatitis B virus vaccine; DTaP = diphtheria and tetanus toxoids and acellular pertussis vaccine; Hib = Haemophilus influenzae type b conjugate vaccine; IPV = inactivated polio vaccine; MMR = live measles, mumps, and rubella viruses vaccine; PCV = pneumococcal conjugate vaccine (Prevnar); Td = adult tetanus toxoid and diphtheria toxoid; VAR = varicella virus vaccine.

Haemophilus Immunization

H influenzae type b Vaccination in Children Immunized Beginning at 2 to 6 Months of Age

Vaccine Product	Total Number of Doses	Regimens
PedvaxHIB (PRP-OMP)	3	2 doses two months apart plus booster at 12-15 months, which must be at least two months after previous dose.

Vaccine Product	Total Number of Doses	Regimens
HibTITER (HbOC), ActHIB (PRP-T), OmniHIB (PRP-T)	4	3 doses two months apart plus booster at 12-15 months which must be at least two months after previous dose. Any vaccine may be used for the booster.

H influenzae type b Vaccination When the Initial Vaccination was Delayed Until 7 Months of Age or Older			
Age at Initiation	Vaccine Product	Total Doses	Regimens
7-11 months	Any vaccine (PedvaxHIB or HibTITER or ActHIB or OmniHIB)	3	2 doses at 2-month intervals plus booster at 12-18 months (at least 2 months after previous dose)
12-14 months	Any vaccine	2	2 doses 2 months apart
15-59 months	Any vaccine	1	Single dose of any product
≥ 5 years	Any vaccine	1	Only recommended for children with chronic illness associated with an increased risk for H flu disease.

Varicella Immunization

Indications for Varicella Immunization:

A. Age 12 to 18 months: One dose of varicella vaccine is recommended for universal immunization for all healthy children who lack a reliable history of varicella.

B. Age 19 months to the 13th birthday: Vaccination of susceptible children is recommended and may be given any time during childhood but before the 13th birthday because of the potential increased severity of natural varicella after this age. Susceptible is defined by either lack of proof of either varicella vaccination or a reliable history of varicella. One dose is recommended.

C. Healthy adolescents and young adults: Healthy adolescents past their 13th birthday who have not been immunized previously and have no history of varicella infection should be immunized against varicella by administration of two doses of vaccine 4 to 8 weeks apart.

D. All susceptible children aged 1 year to 18 years old who are in direct contact with people at high risk for varicella related complications (eg, immunocompromised individuals) and who have not had varicella.

Influenza Immunization

Indications for Influenza Vaccination

A. Targeted high-risk children and adolescents (eg, chronic pulmonary disease including asthma, sickle cell anemia, HIV infection).

B. Other high-risk children and adolescents (eg, diabetes mellitus, chronic renal disease, chronic metabolic disease).

C. Close contacts of high risk patients.

D. Foreign travel if exposure is likely.

Vaccine Administration. Administer in the Fall, usually October 1 - November 15, before the start of the influenza season.

Influenza Immunization Administration			
Age	Vaccine Type	Dosage (mL)	Number of Doses
6-35 months	Split virus only	0.25	1-2*
3-8 years	Split virus only	0.5	1-2*
9-12 years	Split virus only	0.5	1
> 12 years	Whole or split virus	0.5	1
*Two doses administered at least one month apart are recommended for children who are receiving influenza vaccine for the first time.			

Pediatric Symptomatic Care

Antipyretics

Analgesics/Antipyretics:

-Acetaminophen (Tylenol) 10-20 mg/kg/dose PO/PR q4-6h, max 5 doses/day or 80 mg/kg/day or 4 gm/day (whichever is smaller) **OR**

-Acetaminophen dose by age (if weight appropriate for age):

AGE:	mg/dose PO/PR q4-6h prn:
0-3 months	40 mg/dose
4-11 months	80 mg/dose
1-2 year	120 mg/dose
2-3 year	160 mg/dose
4-5 year	240 mg/dose
6-8 year	320 mg/dose
9-10 year	400 mg/dose
11-12 year	480 mg/dose
>12 year	325-650 mg/dose

-Preparations: caplets: 160, 500 mg; caplet, ER: 650 mg; drops: 80 mg/0.8 mL; elixir: 80 mg/2.5 mL, 80 mg/5 mL, 120 mg/5 mL, 160 mg/5 mL, 325 mg/5 mL, 500 mg/15 mL; suppositories: 80, 120, 325, 650 mg; tabs: 325, 500 mg; tabs, chewable: 80, 120, 160 mg.

-Ibuprofen (Motrin, Advil, Nuprin, Medipren, Children's Motrin)

Analgesic: 4-10 mg/kg/dose PO q6-8h prn

Antipyretic: 5-10 mg/kg/dose PO q6-8h.

-Preparations: cap: 200 mg; caplet: 100 mg; oral drops: 40 mg/mL; susp: 100 mg/5 mL; tabs: 100, 200, 300, 400, 600, 800 mg; tabs, chewable: 50, 100 mg.

May cause GI distress, bleeding.

Antitussives, Decongestants, Expectorants, and Antihistamines

Antihistamines:

-Brompheniramine (Dimetane) [elixir: 2 mg/5 mL; tab: 4, 8, 12 mg; tab, SR: 8, 12 mg]

<6 year: 0.5 mg/kg/day PO q6h prn (max 8 mg/day)

6-11 year: 2-4 mg PO q6-8h

≥12 year: 4-8 mg PO q4-6h or 8 mg SR PO q8-12h or 12 mg SR PO q12h (max 24 mg/day).

-Chlorpheniramine (Chlor-Trimeton) [cap, SR: 8, 12 mg; syrup 2mg/5mL; tabs:

4, 8, 12 mg; tab, chew: 2 mg; tab, SR: 8, 12 mg]

2-5 year: 1 mg PO q4-6h prn

6-11 year: 2 mg PO q4-6h prn

$\geq$ 12 year: 4 mg PO q4-6h prn or 8-12 mg SR PO q8-12h

Antitussives (Pure) - Dextromethorphan:

-Benylin DM Cough syrup [syrup: 10 mg/5mL]

-Benylin Pediatric [syrup: 37.5mg/5mL]

-Robitussin Pediatric [syrup: 7.5 mg/5mL]

-Vick's Formula 44 Pediatric Formula [syrup: 3 mg/5mL]

2-5 year: 2.5-5 mg PO q4h prn or 7.5 mg PO q6-8h prn

6-11 year 5-10 mg PO q4h prn or 15 mg PO q6-8h prn

$\geq$12 year: 10-20 mg PO q4h prn or 30 mg PO q6-8h prn.

Expectorants:

-Guaifenesin (Robitussin) [syrup: 100 mg/5 mL]

<2 year: 12 mg/kg/day PO q4-6h prn

2-5 year: 50-100 mg PO q4h prn (max 600 mg/day)

6-11 year: 100-200 mg PO q4h prn (max 1.2 gm/day)

$\geq$12 year: 100-400 mg PO q4h prn (max 2.4 gm/day)

May irritate gastric mucosa; take with large quantities of fluids.

Decongestants:

-Pseudoephedrine (Sudafed, Novafed): [cap: 60 mg; cap, SR: 120, 240 mg; drops: 7.5 mg/0.8 mL; syrup: 15 mg/5 mL, 30 mg/5 mL; tabs: 30, 60 mg].

<2 year: 4 mg/kg/day PO q6h.

2-5 year: 15 mg po q6h.

6-11 year: 30 mg po q6h.

>12 year: 30-60 mg/dose PO q6h or sustained release 120 mg PO q12h or sustained release 240 mg PO q24h.

-Phenylephrine (Neo-synephrine) [nasal drops: 1/4, 1/2, 1%; nasal spray: 1/4, 1/2, 1%].

Children: Use 1/4 % spray or drops, 1-2 drops/spray in each nostril q3-4h.

Adults: Use 1/4-1/2% drops/spray, 1-2 drops/sprays in each nostril q3-4h

Discontinue use after 3 days to avoid rebound congestion.

Combination Products:

-Actifed [per cap or tab or 10 mL syrup: Triprolidine 2.5 mg, Pseudoephedrine 60 mg].

4 month-2 year: 1.25 mL PO q6-8h

2-4 year: 2.5 mL PO q6-8h

4-6 year: 3.75 mL PO q6-8h

6-11year: 5 mL or 1/2 tab PO q6-8h

$\geq$12 year: 10 mL or 1 cap/tab PO q6-8h **OR**

4 mg pseudoephedrine/kg/day PO tid-qid

-Actifed with Codeine cough syrup [syrup/5 mL: Codeine 10 mg, Triprolidine 1.25 mg, Pseudoephedrine 30 mg].

    4 month-2 year: 1.25 mL PO q6-8h
    2-4 year: 2.5 mL PO q6-8h
    4-6 year: 3.75 mL PO q6-8h
    6-11y: 5 mL PO q6-8h
    $\geq$12 year: 10 mL PO q6-8h **OR**
    4 mg pseudoephedrine/kg/day PO tid-qid.
-Dimetane Decongestant [cap/caplet or 10 mL: Brompheniramine 4 mg, Phenylephrine 5 mg].
    6-11 year: 5 mL or 1/2 cap/caplet PO q4-6h
    $\geq$ 12 year: 10 mL or 1 cap/caplet PO q4-6h prn
-Dimetane DX [syrup per 5 mL: Brompheniramine 2 mg, Dextromethorphan 10 mg, Pseudoephedrine 30 mg].
    2-5 years: 2.5 mL PO q4-6h prn
    6-11 years: 5 mL PO q4-6h prn
    $\geq$ 12 years: 10 mL PO q4-6h prn
-PediaCare Cough-Cold Chewable Tablets: [tab, chew: Pseudoephedrine 15 mg, Chlorpheniramine 1 mg, Dextromethorphan 5 mg].
    3-5 year: 1 tab PO q4-6h prn (max 4 tabs/day)
    6-11 year: 2 tabs PO q4-6h (max 8 tabs/day)
    $\geq$12 year: 4 tabs PO q4-6h (max 16 tabs/day)
-PediaCare Cough-Cold Liquid [liquid per 5 mL: Pseudoephedrine 15 mg, Chlorpheniramine 1 mg, Dextromethorphan 5 mg].
    3-5 year: 5 mL PO q6-8h prn
    6-11 year: 10 mL PO q6-8h prn
    $\geq$12 year: 20 mL PO q6-8h prn
-PediaCare Night Rest Cough-Cold Liquid [liquid per 5 mL: Pseudoephedrine 15 mg, Chlorpheniramine 1 mg, Dextromethorphan 7.5 mg].
    3-5 year: 5 mL PO q6-8h prn
    6-11 year: 10 mL PO q6-8h prn
    $\geq$12 year: 20 mL PO q6-8h prn
-Phenergan VC [syrup per 5 mL: Phenylephrine 5 mg, Promethazine 6.25 mg].
    2-5 year: 1.25 mL PO q4-6h prn
    6-11 year: 2.5 mL PO q4-6h prn
    $\geq$12 year: 5 mL PO q4-6h prn
-Phenergan VC with Codeine [per 5 mL: Promethazine 6.25 mg, Codeine 10 mg, Phenylephrine 5 mg].
    2-5 year: 1.25 mL PO q4-6h prn
    6-11 year: 2.5 mL PO q4-6h prn
    $\geq$12 year: 5 mL PO q4-6h prn
    Adults: 5-10 mL q4-6h prn (max 120 mg codeine per day)
-Phenergan with Codeine [syrup per 5 mL: Promethazine 6.25 mg, Codeine 10 mg].
    2-5 year: 1.25 mL PO q4-6h prn
    6-11 year: 2.5 mL PO q4-6h prn

>12 year: 5 mL PO q4-6h prn

Adults: 5-10 mL q4-6h prn (max 120 mg codeine per day)

-Phenergan with Dextromethorphan [syrup per 5 mL: Promethazine 6.25 mg, Dextromethorphan 15 mg].

2-5 year: 1.25 mL PO q4-6h prn

6-11 year: 2.5 mL PO q4-6h prn

>12 year: 5 mL PO q4-6h prn

-Robitussin AC [syrup per 5 mL: Guaifenesin 100 mg, Codeine 10 mg].

6 months-2 year: 1.25-2.5 mL PO q4h prn

2-5 years: 2.5 mL PO q4h prn

6-11 years: 5 mL PO q4h prn

>12 years: 10 mL PO q4-6h prn.

-Robitussin-DAC [syrup per 5 mL: Codeine 10mg, Guaifenesin 100 mg, Pseudoephedrine 30 mg].

2-5 years: 1-1.5 mg/kg/day of codeine PO q4-6h prn (max 30 mg/day)

6-11 years: 5 mL PO q4-6h prn

>12 years: 10 mL PO q4-6h prn

-Robitussin DM [syrup per 5 mL: Guaifenesin 100 mg, Dextromethorphan 10 mg].

2-5 year: 2.5 mL PO q4h prn, max 10 mL/day.

6-11 year: 5 mL PO q4h prn, max 20 mL/day.

>12 year: 10 mL PO q4h prn, max 40 mL/day.

-Robitussin Pediatric Cough and Cold [syrup per 5 mL: Dextromethorphan 7.5mg, Pseudoephedrine 15 mg].

2-5 year: 5 mL PO q4-6h prn.

6-11 year: 10 mL PO q4-6h prn.

>12 year: 15 mL po q4-6h prn.

Maximum four doses daily.

-Rondec drops [drops per 1 mL: Carbinoxamine maleate 2 mg, Pseudo-ephedrine 25 mg].

4-5 mg pseudoephedrine/kg/day PO q6h prn **OR**

1-3 m: 1/4 dropperful (1/4 mL) PO q6h prn

3-6 m: 1/2 dropperful (1/2 mL) PO q6h prn

6-9 m: 3/4 dropperful (0.75 mL) PO q6h prn

9-18 m: 1 dropperful (1 mL) PO q6h prn.

-Rondec syrup [syrup per 5 mL: Pseudoephedrine 60 mg, Carbinoxamine maleate 4 mg].

4-5 mg pseudoephedrine/kg/day PO q6h prn.

-Rondec DM drops [drops per mL: Carbinoxamine maleate 2 mg, Pseudoephedrine 25 mg, Dextromethorphan 4 mg].

4-5 mg pseudoephedrine/kg/day PO q6h prn **OR**

1-3 m: 1/4 dropperful (1/4 mL) PO q6h prn

3-6 m: 1/2 dropperful (1/2 mL) PO q6h prn

6-9 m: 3/4 dropperful (0.75 mL) PO q6h prn

9-18 m: 1 dropperful (1 mL) PO q6h prn.

-Rondec DM syrup [syrup per 5 mL: Carbinoxamine maleate 4 mg, Pseudoephedrine 60 mg, Dextromethorphan 15 mg].

  4-5 mg pseudoephedrine/kg/day PO q6h prn.

-Ryna Liquid [liquid per 5 mL: Chlorpheniramine 2 mg; Pseudoephedrine 30 mg].

  6-11 years: 5 mL PO q6h prn.

  $\geq$12 year: 10 mL PO q6h prn.

-Ryna-C [liquid per 5 mL: Chlorpheniramine 2 mg, Codeine 10 mg, Pseudoephedrine 30 mg].

  4-5 mg/kg/day of pseudoephedrine component PO q6h prn

-Ryna-CS [liquid per 5 mL: Codeine 10 mg, Guaifenesin 100 mg, Pseudoephedrine 30 mg].

  4-5 mg pseudoephedrine/kg/day PO q6h prn

-Rynatan Pediatric [susp per 5 mL: Chlorpheniramine 2 mg, Phenylephrine 5 mg, Pyrilamine 12.5 mg].

  2-5 year: 2.5-5 mL PO bid prn

  6-11 year: 5-10 mL PO bid prn

  $\geq$12 year: 10-15 mL PO bid prn

-Tylenol Cold Multi-Symptom Plus Cough Liquid, Children's [liquid per 5 mL: Acetaminophen 160 mg, Chlorpheniramine 1 mg, Pseudoephedrine 15 mg].

  2-5 year: 5 mL PO q4h prn

  6-11 year: 10 mL PO q4h prn

  $\geq$12 year: 20 mL po q4h prn

  Maximum four doses daily.

-Tylenol Cold Plus Cough Chewable Tablet, Children's [tab, chew: Acetaminophen 80 mg, Chlorpheniramine 0.5 mg, Dextromethorphan 2.5 mg, Pseudoephedrine 7.5 mg].

  2-5 year: 2 tabs PO q4h prn

  6-11 year: 4 tabs PO q4h prn

  $\geq$12 year: 4 tabs PO q4h prn

  Maximum four doses daily.

-Vick's Children's NyQuil Night-time Cough/Cold [liquid per 5 mL: Chlorpheniramine 0.67 mg; Dextromethorphan 5 mg, Pseudoephedrine 10 mg].

  6-11 year: 15 mL PO q6-8h prn

  $\geq$12 year: 30 mL PO q6-8h prn

-Vick's Pediatric Formula 44D [liquid per 5 mL: Dextromethorphan 5 mg, Pseudoephedrine 10 mg].

  2-5 year: 3.75 mL PO q6h prn

  6-11 year: 7.5 mL po q6h prn

  $\geq$12 year: 15 mL PO q6h prn

-Vick's Pediatric Formula 44E [syrup per 5 mL: Dextromethorphan 3.3 mg, Guaifenesin 33.3 mg].

  2-5 year: 5 mL PO q4h prn

6-11 year: 10 mL PO q4h prn

≥12 year: 15 mL po q4h prn

-Vick's Pediatric Formula 44M Multi-Symptom Cough and Cold Liquid [liquid per 5 mL: Chlorpheniramine 0.67 mg, Dextromethorphan 5 mg, Pseudoephedrine 10 mg].

2-5 year: 7.5 mL PO q6h prn

6-11 year: 15 mL PO q6h prn

≥12 year: 30 mL PO q6h prn

Analgesia and Sedation

Analgesics/Anesthetic Agents:

-Acetaminophen (Tylenol) 10-15 mg/kg PO/PR q4-6h prn (see page 17 for detailed list of available products)

-Acetaminophen/Codeine [per 5 mL: Acetaminophen 120 mg, Codeine 12 mg; tabs: Tylenol #2: 15 mg codeine/300 mg acetaminophen; #3: 30 mg codeine/300 mg acetaminophen; #4: 60 mg codeine/300 mg acetaminophen]

0.5-1.0 mg codeine/kg/dose PO q4h prn.

-Acetaminophen/Hydrocodone [elixir per 5 mL: hydrocodone 2.5 mg, acetaminophen 167 mg]

Tab:

Lortab 2.5/500: Hydrocodone 2.5 mg, acetaminophen 500 mg

Lortab 5/500 and Vicodin: Hydrocodone 5 mg, acetaminophen 500 mg

Lortab 7.5/500: Hydrocodone 7.5 mg, acetaminophen 500 mg

Vicodin ES: Hydrocodone 7.5 mg, acetaminophen 750 mg

Lortab 10/500: Hydrocodone 10 mg, acetaminophen 500 mg

Lortab 10/650: Hydrocodone 10 mg, acetaminophen 650 mg

Children: 0.6 mg hydrocodone/kg/day PO q6-8h prn

<2 year: do not exceed 1.25 mg/dose

2-12 year: do not exceed 5 mg/dose

>12 year: do not exceed 10 mg/dose

-ELAMax [lidocaine 4% cream (liposomal): 5, 30 gm]

Apply 10-60 minutes prior to procedure. Occlusive dressing is optional. Available OTC.

-EMLA cream (eutectic mixture of local anesthetics) [cream: 2.5% lidocaine and 2.5% prilocaine: 5, 30 gm; transdermal disc]. Apply and cover with occlusive dressing at least 1 hour (max 4 hours) prior to procedure.

-Fentanyl 1-2 mcg/kg IV q1-2h prn or 1-3 mcg/kg/hr continuous IV infusion.

-Hydromorphone (Dilaudid) 0.015 mg/kg IV/IM/SC q3-4h or

0.0075 mg/kg/hr continuous IV infusion titrated as necessary for pain relief or 0.03-0.08 mg/kg PO q6h prn.

-Ketamine 4 mg/kg IM or 0.5-1 mg/kg IV. Onset for IV administration is 30 seconds, duration is 5-15 minutes.

-Lidocaine, buffered: Add sodium bicarbonate 1 mEq/mL 1 part to 9 parts lidocaine 1% for local infiltration (eg, 2 mL lidocaine 1% and 0.22 mL sodium bicarbonate 1 mEq/mL) to raise the pH of the lidocaine to neutral and decrease the "sting" of subcutaneous lidocaine.

-Meperidine (Demerol) 1 mg/kg IV/IM q2-3h prn pain.

-Morphine 0.05-0.1 mg/kg IV q2-4h prn or 0.02-0.06 mg/kg/hr continuous IV infusion or 0.1-0.15 mg/kg IM/SC q3-4h or 0.2-0.5 mg/kg PO q4-6h.

Sedation:
Fentanyl and Midazolam Sedation:

-Fentanyl 1 mcg/kg IV slowly, may repeat to total of 3 mcg/kg **AND**

-Midazolam (Versed) 0.05-0.1 mg/kg slow IV [inj: 1 mg/mL, 5 mg/mL].

Have reversal agents available: naloxone 0.1 mg/kg (usual max 2 mg) IM/IV for fentanyl reversal and flumazenil 0.01 mg/kg (usual max 5 mg) IM/IV for midazolam reversal.

Benzodiazepines:

-Diazepam (Valium) 0.2-0.5 mg/kg/dose PO/PR or 0.05-0.2 mg/kg/dose IM/IV, max 10 mg.

-Lorazepam (Ativan) 0.05-0.1 mg/kg/dose IM/IV/PO, max 4 mg.

-Midazolam (Versed) 0.08-0.2 mg/kg/dose IM/IV over 10-20 min, max 5 mg; or 0.2-0.4 mg/kg/dose PO x 1, max 15 mg, 30-45 min prior to procedure; or 0.2 mg/kg intranasal (using 5 mg/mL injectable solution, insert into nares with needleless tuberculin syringe.)

Phenothiazines:

-Promethazine (Phenergan) 0.5-1 mg/kg/dose IM or slow IV over 20 min, max 50 mg/dose.

-Chlorpromazine (Thorazine) 0.5-1 mg/kg/dose IM or slow IV over 20min, max 50 mg/dose.

Antihistamines:

-Diphenhydramine (Benadryl) 1 mg/kg/dose IV/IM/PO, max 50 mg.

-Hydroxyzine (Vistaril) 0.5-1 mg/kg/dose IM/PO, max 50 mg.

Barbiturates:

-Methohexital (Brevital)

    IM: 5-10 mg/kg

    IV: 1-2 mg/kg

    PR: 25 mg/kg (max 500 mg/dose)

-Thiopental (Pentothal): Sedation, rectal: 5-10 mg/kg; seizures, IV: 2-3 mg/kg

Other Sedatives:

-Chloral hydrate 25-100 mg/kg/dose PO/PR (max 1.5 gm/dose), allow 30 min for absorption.

Nonsteroidal Anti-Inflammatory Drugs (NSAIDS):

-Ibuprofen (Motrin, Advil, Nuprin, Medipren, Children's Motrin)

    Anti-inflammatory: 30-50 mg/kg/day PO q6h, max 2400 mg/day.

[cap: 200 mg; caplet: 100 mg; oral drops: 40 mg/mL; susp: 100 mg/5 mL;
tabs: 100, 200, 300, 400, 600, 800 mg; tabs, chewable: 50, 100 mg].
-Ketorolac (Toradol)
Single dose: 0.4-1 mg/kg IV/IM (max 30 mg/dose IV, 60 mg/dose IM)
Multiple doses: 0.4-0.5 mg/kg IV/IM q6h prn (max 30 mg/dose)
[inj: 15 mg/mL, 30 mg/mL].
Do not use for more than three days because of risk of GI bleed.
-Naproxen (Naprosyn)
Analgesia: 5-7 mg/kg/dose PO q8-12h
Inflammatory disease: 10-15 mg/kg/day PO q12h, max 1000 mg/day
[susp: 125 mg/5mL; tab: 250, 375, 500 mg; tab, DR: 375, 500 mg
-Naproxen sodium (Aleve, Anaprox, Naprelan)
Analgesia: 5-7 mg/kg/dose PO q8-12h
Inflammatory disease: 10-15 mg/kg/day PO q12h, max 1000 mg/day
[tab: 220, 275, 550 mg; tab, ER: 375, 500, 750 mg]. Naproxen sodium
220 mg = 200 mg base.

Antiemetics

-Chlorpromazine (Thorazine)
0.25-1 mg/kg/dose slow IV over 20 min/IM/PO q4-8h prn, max 50 mg/dose
[inj: 25 mg/mL,; oral concentrate 30 mg/mL; supp: 25,100 mg; syrup: 10
mg/5 mL; tabs: 10, 25, 50, 100, 200 mg].
-Diphenhydramine (Benadryl)
1 mg/kg/dose IM/IV/PO q6h prn, max 50 mg/dose
[caps: 25, 50 mg; inj: 10 mg/mL, 50 mg/mL; liquid: 12.5 mg/5 mL; tabs: 25,
50 mg].
-Dimenhydrinate (Dramamine)
≥12 years: 5 mg/kg/day IM/IV/PO q6h prn, max 300 mg/day
Not recommended in <12y due to high incidence of extrapyramidal side
effects.
[cap: 50 mg; inj: 50 mg/mL; liquid 12.5 mg/4 mL; tab: 50 mg; tab, chew:
50mg].
-Prochlorperazine (Compazine)
≥12 years: 0.1-0.15 mg/kg/dose IM, max 10 mg/dose or 5-10 mg PO q6-8h,
max 40 mg/day **OR** 5-25 mg PR q12h, max 50 mg/day
Not recommended in <12y due to high incidence of extrapyramidal side
effects
[caps, SR: 10, 15, 30 mg; inj: 5 mg/mL; supp: 2.5, 5, 25 mg; syrup: 5 mg/5
mL; tabs: 5, 10, 25 mg].
-Promethazine (Phenergan)
0.25-1 mg/kg/dose PO/IM/IV over 20 min or PR q4-6h prn, max 50 mg/dose
[inj: 25,50 mg/mL; supp: 12.5, 25, 50 mg; syrup 6.25 mg/5 mL, 25 mg/5 mL;

tabs: 12.5, 25, 50 mg].
-Trimethobenzamide (Tigan)
   15 mg/kg/day IM/PO/PR q6-8h, max 100 mg/dose if <13.6 kg or 200 mg/dose if 13.6-41kg.
   [caps: 100, 250 mg; inj: 100 mg/mL; supp: 100, 200 mg].

Post-Operative Nausea and Vomiting:
-Ondansetron (Zofran) 0.1 mg/kg IV x 1, max 4 mg.
-Droperidol (Inapsine) 0.01-0.05 mg/kg IV/IM q4-6h prn, max 5 mg [inj: 2.5 mg/mL].

Chemotherapy-Induced Nausea:
-Dexamethasone
   10 mg/m^2/dose (max 20 mg) IV x 1, then 5 mg/m^2/dose (max 10 mg) IV q6h prn
   [inj: 4 mg/mL, 10 mg/mL]
-Dronabinol (Marinol)
   5 mg/m^2/dose PO 1-3 hrs prior to chemotherapy, then q4h prn afterwards.
   May titrate up in 2.5 mg/m^2/dose increments to max of 15 mg/m^2/dose.
   [cap: 2.5, 5, 10 mg]
-Granisetron (Kytril)
   10-20 mcg/kg IV given just prior to chemotherapy (single dose) [inj: 1 mg/mL]
   Adults (oral) 1 mg PO bid or 2 mg PO qd [tab: 1 mg]
-Metoclopramide (Reglan)
   0.5-1 mg/kg/dose IV q6h prn.
   Pretreatment with diphenhydramine 1 mg/kg IV is recommended to decrease the risk of extrapyramidal reactions.
   [inj: 5 mg/mL]
-Ondansetron (Zofran)
   0.15 mg/kg/dose IV 30 minutes before chemotherapy and repeated 4 hr and 8 hr later (total of 3 doses) **OR**
   0.3 mg/kg/dose IV x 1 30 minutes before chemotherapy **OR**
   0.45 mg/kg/day as a continuous IV infusion **OR**
   Oral:
   <0.3 m^2: 1 mg PO three times daily
   0.3-0.6 m^2: 2 mg PO three times daily
   0.6-1 m^2: 3 mg PO three times daily
   >1 m^2: 4 mg PO three times daily **OR**
   4-11 year: 4 mg PO three times daily
   >11 year: 8 mg PO three times daily
   [inj: 2 mg/mL; oral soln: 4mg/5 mL; tab: 4, 8, 24 mg; tab, orally disintegrating: 4, 8 mg]

Cardiovascular Disorders

Pediatric Advanced Life Support

I. **Cardiopulmonary assessment**
   A. **Airway (A) assessment**. The airway should be assessed and cleared.
   B. **Breathing (B) assessment** determines the respiratory rate, respiratory effort, breath sounds (air entry), and skin color. A respiratory rate of less than 10 or greater than 60 is a sign of impending respiratory failure.
   C. **Circulation © assessment** should quantify the heart rate and pulse. In infants, chest compressions should be initiated if the heart rate is less than 80 beats/minute (bpm). In children, chest compressions should be initiated if the heart rate is less than 60 bpm.

II. **Respiratory failure**
   A. An open airway should be established. Bag-valve-mask ventilation should be initiated if the respiratory rate is less than 10. Intubation is performed if prolonged ventilation is required. Matching the endotracheal tube to the size of the nares or fifth finger provides an estimate of tube size.

Intubation			
Age	ETT	Laryngoscope Blade	NG Tube Size
Premature	2.0-2.5	0	8
Newborn >2 kg	3.0-3.5	1	10
Infant	3.5-4.0	1	10
12 months	4.0-4.5	1.5	12
36 months	4.5-5.0	2	12-14
6 year	5.0-5.5	2	14-16
10 year	6.0-6.5	2	16-18
Adolescent	.0-7.5	3	18-20
Adult	7.5-8.0	3	20

Uncuffed ET tube in children <8 years.
Straight laryngoscope blade if <6-10 years; curved blade if older.

   B. Vascular access should be obtained. Gastric decompression with a nasogastric or orogastric tube is necessary in endotracheally intubated children and in children receiving bag-valve-mask ventilation.

III. **Shock**

A. If the child is in shock, oxygen administration and monitoring are followed by initiation of vascular access. Crystalloid (normal saline or lactated Ringer's) solutions are used for rapid fluid boluses of 20 mL/kg over less than 20 minutes until the shock is resolved.

B. Shock secondary to traumatic blood loss may require blood replacement if perfusion parameters have not normalized after a total of 40 to 60 mL/kg of crystalloid has been administered.

C. Children in septic shock and cardiogenic shock should initially receive crystalloid solution (boluses of 20 mL/kg). Epinephrine should be considered if septic or cardiogenic shock persists after intravenous volume has been repleted (repletion requires 40 to 60 mL/kg of crystalloid).

IV. **Cardiopulmonary failure**

A. Oxygen is delivered at a concentration of 100%.

B. Intubation and foreign body removal are completed. If signs of shock persist, crystalloid replacement is initiated with boluses of 20 mL/kg over less than 20 minutes. Inotropic agents are added if hypotension persists.

Inotropic Agents Used in Resuscitation of Children		
Agent	**Intravenous dosage**	**Indications**
Epinephrine	0.1 to 1.0 µg/kg/minute (continuous infusion)	Symptomatic bradycardia, shock (cardiogenic, septic, anaphylactic), hypotension
Dopamine	2 to 5 µg/kg/minute (continuous infusion) 10 to 20 µg/kg/minute (continuous infusion)	Low dose: improve renal and splanchnic blood flow. High dose: useful in the treatment of hypotension and shock in the presence of adequate intravascular volume
Dobutamine	2 to 20 µg/kg/minute (continuous infusion)	Normotensive cardiogenic shock

V. **Dysrhythmias**

A. **Bradycardia**

1. Bradycardia is the most common dysrhythmia in children. Initial management is ventilation and oxygenation. Chest compressions should be initiated if the heart rate is <60 bpm in a child or <80 bpm in an infant.

2. If these measures do not restore the heart rate, epinephrine is

administered. Intravenous or intraosseous epinephrine is given in a dose of 0.1 mL/kg of the 1:10,000 concentration (0.01 mg/kg). Endotracheal tube epinephrine is given as a dose of 0.1 mL/kg of the 1:1,000 concentration (0.1 mg/kg) diluted to a final volume of 3-5 mL in normal saline. This dose may be repeated every three to five minutes.

3. Atropine may be tried if multiple doses of epinephrine are unsuccessful. Atropine is given in a dose of 0.2 mL/kg IV/IO/ET of the 1:10,000 concentration (0.02 mg/kg. The minimum dose is 0.1 mg; the maximum single dose is 0.5 mg for a child and 1 mg for an adolescent. Endotracheal tube administration of atropine should be further diluted to a final volume of 3-5 mL in normal saline.

4. Pacing may be attempted if drug therapy has failed.

B. Asystole

1. Epinephrine is the drug of choice for asystole. The initial dose of intravenous or intraosseous epinephrine is given as 0.1 mL/kg of the 1:10,000 concentration of epinephrine (0.01 mg/kg). Endotracheal tube administration of epinephrine is given as 0.1 mL/kg of the 1:1,000 concentration of epinephrine (0.1 mg/kg), diluted to a final volume of 3-5 mL in normal saline.

2. Subsequent doses of epinephrine are administered every three to five minutes at 0.1 mL/kg IV/IO/ET of the 1:1,000 concentration (0.1 mg/kg).

C. Supraventricular tachycardia

1. Supraventricular tachycardia presents with a heart rate >220 beats/minute in infants and >180 beats/minute in children. Supraventricular tachycardia is the most common dysrhythmia in the first year of life.

2. **Stable children with no signs of respiratory compromise or shock and a normal blood pressure**
   a. Initiate 100% oxygen and cardiac monitoring.
   b. Administer adenosine 0.1 mg/kg (max 6 mg) by rapid intravenous push. The dose of adenosine may be doubled to 0.2 mg/kg (max 12 mg) and repeated if supraventricular tachycardia is not converted.
   c. **Verapamil (Calan)** may be used; however, it is contraindicated under one year; in congestive heart failure or myocardial depression; in children receiving beta-adrenergic blockers; and in the presence of a possible bypass tract (ie, Wolff-Parkinson-White syndrome). Dose is 0.1-0.3 mg/kg/dose (max 5 mg) IV; may repeat dose in 30 minutes prn (max 10 mg).

3. **Supraventricular tachycardia in unstable child with signs of shock**: Administer synchronized cardioversion at 0.5 joules/kg. If supraventricular tachycardia persists, cardioversion is repeated at

double the dose: 1.0 J/kg.

D. Ventricular tachycardia with palpable pulse

1. A palpable pulse with heart rate $\geq$120 bpm with a wide QRS (>0.08 seconds) is present. Initiate cardiac monitoring, administer oxygen and ventilate.
2. If vascular access is available, administer a lidocaine bolus of 1 mg/kg; if successful, begin lidocaine infusion at 20-50 µg/kg/minute.
3. If ventricular tachycardia persists, perform synchronized cardioversion using 0.5 J/kg.
4. If ventricular tachycardia persists, repeat synchronized cardioversion using 1.0 J/kg.
5. If ventricular tachycardia persists, administer a lidocaine bolus of 1.0 mg/kg, and begin lidocaine infusion at 20-50 µg/kg/min.
6. Repeat synchronized cardioversion as indicated.

E. Ventricular fibrillation and pulseless ventricular tachycardia

1. Apply cardiac monitor, administer oxygen, and ventilate.
2. Perform defibrillation using 2 J/kg. Do not delay defibrillation.
3. If ventricular fibrillation persists, perform defibrillation using 4 J/kg.
4. If ventricular fibrillation persists, perform defibrillation using 4 J/kg.
5. If ventricular fibrillation persists, perform intubation, continue CPR, and obtain vascular access. Administer epinephrine, 0.1 mL/kg of 1:10,000 IV or IO (0.01 mg/kg); or 0.1 mL/kg of 1:1000 ET (0.1 mg/kg).
6. If ventricular fibrillation persists, perform defibrillation using 4 J/kg.
7. If ventricular fibrillation persists, administer lidocaine 1 mg/kg IV or IO, or 2 mg/kg ET.
8. If ventricular fibrillation persists, perform defibrillation using 4 J/kg.
9. If ventricular fibrillation persists, continue epinephrine, 0.1 mg/kg IV/IO/ET, 0.1 mL/kg of 1:1,000; administer every 3 to 5 minutes.
10. If ventricular fibrillation persists, alternate defibrillation (4 J/kg) with lidocaine and epinephrine. Consider bretylium 5 mg/kg IV first dose, 10 mg/kg IV second dose.

F. Pulseless electrical activity is uncommon in children. It usually occurs secondary to hypoxemia, hypovolemia, hypothermia, hypoglycemia, hyperkalemia, cardiac tamponade, tension pneumothorax, severe acidosis or drug overdose. Successful resuscitation depends on treatment of the underlying etiology.

1. The initial dose of IV or IO epinephrine is given in a dose of 0.1 mL/kg of the 1:10,000 concentration (0.01 mg/kg). Endotracheal epinephrine is given as a dose of 0.1 mL/kg of the 1:1,000 concentration (0.1 mg/kg) diluted to a final volume of 3-5 mL in normal saline.
2. Subsequent doses are administered every three to five minutes as 0.1 mL/kg of the 1:1,000 concentration IV/IO/ET (0.1 mg/kg).

VI. Serum glucose concentration should be determined in all children undergoing resuscitation. Glucose replacement is provided with 25% dextrose in water, 2 to 4 mL/kg (0.5 to 1 g/kg) IV over 20 to 30 minutes for hypoglycemia. In neonates, 10% dextrose in water, 5 to 10 mL/kg (0.5 to 1 g/kg), is used.

Congestive Heart Failure

1. **Admit to:**
2. **Diagnosis:** Congestive Heart Failure.
3. **Condition:**
4. **Vital signs:** Call MD if:
5. **Activity:**
6. **Nursing:** Daily weights, inputs and outputs .
7. **Diet:** Low-salt diet.
8. **IV Fluids:**
9. **Special Medications:**
   -Oxygen 2-4 L/min by NC.
   -Furosemide (Lasix) 1 mg/kg/dose IV/IM/PO q6-12h prn, max 80 mg PO, 40 mg IV; may increase to 2 mg/kg/dose IV/IM/PO.
   [inj: 10 mg/mL; oral liquid: 10 mg/mL, 40 mg/5 mL; tabs: 20, 40, 80 mg] **OR**
   -Bumetanide (Bumex) 0.015-0.1 mg/kg PO/IV/IM q12-24h, max 10 mg/day
   [inj: 0.25 mg/mL; tabs: 0.5, 1, 2 mg].

Digoxin:
   -Obtain a baseline ECG, serum electrolytes (potassium), and serum creatinine before administration.
   Initial digitalization is given over 24 hours in three divided doses: 1/2 total digitalizing dose (TDD) at time 0 hours, 1/4 TDD at 8-12 hours, and 1/4 TDD 8-12 hours later.
   Maintenance therapy is then started.

Total Digitalizing Dose

	PO	IV
Premature infant	20-30 mcg/kg	10-30 mcg/kg
Full term newborn (0-2 weeks)	30 mcg/kg	20-25 mcg/kg
2 weeks-2 year	40-50 mcg/kg	30-40 mcg/kg
2-10 year	30-40 mcg/kg	25-30 mcg/kg
>10 year	0.75-1.5 mg	10 mcg/kg (max 1 mg)

Maintenance digoxin dose

	PO	**IV**
Preterm neonate	4-10 mcg/kg/day	4-9 mcg/kg/day
Term neonate (0-2 weeks)	6-10 mcg/kg/day	6-8 mcg/kg/day
2 weeks - 2 year	10-12 mcg/kg/day	8-10 mcg/kg/day
2-10 year	8-10 mcg/kg/day	6-8 mcg/kg/day
>10 year	5 mcg/kg/day	2-3 mcg/kg/day
Adult	0.125-0.5 mg/day	0.1-0.4 mg/day

Divide bid if <10 years or qd if >10 years.

[caps: 50, 100, 200 mcg; elixir: 50 mcg/mL; inj: 100 mcg/mL, 250 mcg/mL; tabs: 0.125, 0.25, 0.5 mg].

Other Agents:

-Dopamine (Intropin) 2-20 mcg/kg/min continuous IV infusion.

-Dobutamine (Dobutrex) 2-20 mcg/kg/min continuous IV infusion, max of 40 mcg/kg/min.

-Nitroglycerin 0.5 mcg/kg/min continuous IV infusion, may increase by 1 mcg/kg q20min; usual max 5 mcg/kg/min.

-Captopril (Capoten)

Neonates: 0.05-0.1 mg/kg/dose PO q6-8h

Infants: 0.15-0.3 mg/kg/dose PO q8h.

Children: 0.5 mg/kg/dose PO q6-12h. Titrate as needed up to max of 6 mg/kg/day

[tabs: 12.5, 25, 50,100 mg]. Tablets can be crushed and made into extemporaneous suspension.

-KCl 1-4 mEq/kg/day PO q6-24h.

10. Extras and X-rays: CXR PA and LAT, ECG, echocardiogram.

11. Labs: ABG, SMA 7, Mg, Ca, CBC, iron studies, digoxin level, UA.

Atrial Fibrillation

1. **Admit to:**
2. **Diagnosis:** Atrial fibrillation.
3. **Condition:**
4. **Vital signs:** Call MD if:
5. **Activity:**
6. **Nursing:**
7. **Diet:**
8. **IV Fluids:**

9. Special Medications:

Cardioversion (if unstable or refractory to drug treatment):

1. If unstable, synchronized cardioversion using 0.5 J/kg. In stable patient with atrial fibrillation, consider starting quinidine or procainamide 24-48h prior to cardioversion.

   -Quinidine gluconate 2-10 mg/kg/dose IV q3-6h.

   -Procainamide: loading dose: 3-6 mg/kg IV over 5 min (max 100 mg), may repeat every 5-10 minutes to max of 15 mg/kg (max 500 mg). Maintenance: 20-80 mcg/kg/min continuous IV infusion (max 2 gm/24 hrs).

2. Midazolam (Versed) 0.1 mg/kg (max 5 mg) IV over 2 min, repeat prn until amnesic.

3. Synchronized cardioversion using 0.5 J/kg. Increase stepwise by 0.5 J/kg if initial dosage fails to convert the patient. Consider esophageal overdrive pacing.

Digoxin Rate Control:

Initial digitalization is given over 24 hours in three divided doses: 1/2 total digitalizing dose (TDD) at time 0 hours, 1/4 TDD at 8-12 hours, and 1/4 TDD 8-12 hours later. Maintenance therapy is then started.

Total Digitalizing Dose

	PO	IV
Premature infant	20-30 mcg/kg	10-30 mcg/kg
Full term newborn (0-2 weeks)	30 mcg/kg	20-25 mcg/kg
2 week-2 year	40-50 mcg/kg	30-40 mcg/kg
2-10 year	30-40 mcg/kg	25-30 mcg/kg
>10 year	0.75-1.5 mg	10 mcg/kg (max 1 mg)

Maintenance Digoxin Dose

	PO	IV
Preterm neonate	4-10 mcg/kg/day	4-9 mcg/kg/day
Term neonate (0-2 weeks	6-10 mcg/kg/day	6-8 mcg/kg/day
2 weeks - 2 year	10-12 mcg/kg/day	8-10 mcg/kg/day
2-10 year	8-10 mcg/kg/day	6-8 mcg/kg/day
>10 year	5 mcg/kg/day	2-3 mcg/kg/day

Divide bid if <10 years or qd if >10 years.

[caps: 50, 100, 200 mcg; elixir: 50 mcg/mL; inj: 100 mcg/mL, 250 mcg/mL; tabs: 0.125, 0.25, 0.5 mg].

Other Rate-Control Agents:

-Propranolol 0.01-0.1 mg/kg slow IV push over 10 minutes, repeat q6-8h prn (max 1 mg/dose) or 0.5-4 mg/kg/day PO q6-8h (max 60 mg/day)

[inj: 1 mg/mL; oral solutions: 4 mg/mL, 8 mg/mL; oral concentrate: 80 mg/mL; tabs: 10, 20, 40, 60, 80, 90 mg].

Pharmacologic Conversion (after rate control):
-Procainamide (Pronestyl): Loading dose of 2-6 mg/kg/dose IV over 5 min, then 20-80 mcg/kg/min IV infusion (max 100 mg/dose or 2 gm/24h). Oral maintenance: 15-50 mg/kg/day PO q3-6h (max 4 gm/day).
[caps: 250, 375, 500 mg; inj: 100 mg/mL, 500 mg/mL; tabs: 250, 375, 500 mg; tabs, SR: 250, 500, 750, 1000 mg].

10. **Extras and X-rays:** Portable CXR, ECG, echocardiogram.
11. **Labs:** CBC, SMA 7, Mg, Ca, UA, ABG. Serum drug levels.

Hypertensive Emergencies

1. **Admit to:**
2. **Diagnosis:** Hypertensive Emergency.
3. **Condition:**
4. **Vital signs:** Call MD if systolic BP >150 mm Hg, diastolic bp >90 mm Hg, MAP >120 mm Hg.
5. **Activity:**
6. **Nursing:** BP q1h, ECG, daily weights, inputs and outputs.
7. **Diet:**
8. **IV Fluids:**
9. **Special Medications:**
    -Nitroprusside (Nipride) 0.5-10 mcg/kg/min continuous IV infusion. Titrate to desired blood pressure. Cyanide and thiocyanate toxicity may develop with prolonged use or in renal impairment.
    -Labetalol (Trandate) 0.2 mg/kg (max 20 mg) IV over 2 min or 0.4-1 mg/kg/hr continuous infusion.
    -Enalaprilat (Vasotec IV) 5-10 mcg/kg/dose IV q8-24h prn.
    -Nifedipine (Adalat, Procardia): 0.25-0.5 mg/kg/dose PO (max 10 mg/dose) q4h prn [trade name capsules: 10 mg/0.34 mL, 20 mg/0.45 mL.
10. **Extras and X-rays:** CXR, ECG, renal Doppler and ultrasound. Hypertensive intravenous pyelography.
11. **Labs:** CBC, SMA 7, BUN, creatinine, UA with micro. Urine specific gravity, thyroid panel, 24h urine for metanephrines; ANA, complement, ASO titer; toxicology screen.

Pulmonary Disorders

Asthma

1. **Admit to:**
2. **Diagnosis:** Exacerbation of asthma.
3. **Condition:**
4. **Vital signs:** Call MD if:
5. **Activity:**
6. **Nursing:** Pulse oximeter, measure peak flow rate in older patients.
7. **Diet:**
8. **IV Fluids:** D5 1/4 NS or D5 1/2 NS at maintenance rate.
9. **Special Medications:**
   -Oxygen humidified prn, 1-6 L/min by NC or 25-80% by mask, keep sat >92%.

Aerosolized and Nebulized Beta-$_2$agonists:
   -Albuterol (Ventolin [using 0.5% = 5 mg/mL soln]) nebulized 0.2-0.5 mL in
      2 mL NS q1-4h and prn; may also be given by continuous aerosol.
      [soln for inhalation: 0.83 mg/3 mL unit dose; 5 mg/mL 20 mL multidose
      bulk bottle]
   -Albuterol (Ventolin, Proventil) 2 puffs q1-6h prn with spacer and mask.
      [capsule for inhalation (Rotacaps) using Rotahaler inhalation device: 200
      mcg; MDI: 90 mcg/puff, 200 puffs/17 gm]
   -Levalbuterol (Xopenex)
      2-11 years: 0.16-1.25 mg nebulized
      $\geq$12 years: 0.63-1.25mg nebulized q6-8h
      [soln for inhalation: 0.63 mg/3 mL, 1.25 mg/3 mL]. Levalbuterol 0.63 mg
      is comparable to albuterol 2.5 mg.
   -Salmeterol (Serevent) >4 years: 2 puffs bid. Not indicated for acute
      treatment. [Serevent Diskus: 50 mcg/puff; MDI: 21 mcg/puff, 60
      puffs/6.5gm or 120 puffs/13 gm]
   -Formoterol (Foradil): $\geq$5 years: 12 mcg capsule aerosolized using dry powder
      inhaler bid. [capsule for aerosolization: 12 mcg]
   -Metaproterenol (Alupent, Metaprel)
      > 12 years: 2-3 puffs q3-4h prn, max 12 puffs/24 hrs. [MDI: 0.65 mg/puff]
   -Racemic epinephrine (2.25% soln) 0.05 mL/kg/dose (max 0.5 mL) in 2-3 mL
      saline nebulized q1-6h.

Intravenous Beta-$_2$ Agonist:
   -Terbutaline (Brethaire, Brethine, Bricanyl)
      Loading dose: 2-10 mcg/kg IV
      Maintenance continuous IV infusion: 0.08-6 mcg/kg/min
      Monitor heart rate and blood pressure closely.
      [inj: 1 mg/mL]

Corticosteroid (systemic) Pulse Therapy:
-Prednisolone 1-2 mg/kg/day PO q12-24h x 3-5 days
[syrup: 5 mg/5 mL; Orapred 20.2 mg/5mL; Prelone 15 mg/5 mL] **OR**
-Prednisone 1-2 mg/kg/day PO q12-24h x 3-5 days
[oral solution: 1 mg/mL, 5 mg/mL; tabs: 1, 2, 5, 10, 20, 50 mg] **OR**
-Methylprednisolone (Solu-Medrol) 2 mg/kg/dose IV/IM q6h x 1-4 doses, then
0.5-1 mg/kg/dose IV/IM q6h x 3-5 days.

Aminophylline and theophylline:
-Therapeutic range 10-20 mcg/mL. Concomitant drugs (eg, erythromycin or
carbamazepine) may increase serum theophylline levels by decreasing
drug metabolism.
-Aminophylline loading dose 5-6 mg/kg **total** body weight IV over 20-30 min
[1 mg/kg of aminophylline will raise serum level by 2 mcg/mL].
-Aminophylline maintenance as continuous IV infusion (based on ideal body
weight)
1-6 month: 0.5 mg/kg/hr
6-12 month: 0.6-0.75 mg/kg/hr
1-10 year: 1.0 mg/kg/hr
10-16 year: 0.75-0.9 mg/kg/hr
>16 year: 0.7 mg/kg/hr **OR**
-Theophylline PO maintenance
80% of total daily maintenance IV aminophylline dose in 2-4 doses/day
OR
1-6 month: 9.6 mg/kg/day.
6-12 month: 11.5-14.4 mg/kg/day.
1-10 year: 19.2 mg/kg/day.
10-16 year: 14.4-17.3 mg/kg/day.
>16 year: 10 mg/kg/day.
-Give theophylline as sustained-release theophylline preparation: q8-12h or
liquid immediate release: q6h.
-Slo-Phyllin Gyrocaps, may open caps and sprinkle on food [60, 125, 250 mg
caps] q8-12h
-Slobid Gyrocaps, may open caps and sprinkle on food [50, 75, 100, 125,
200, 300 mg caps] q8-12h
-Theophylline oral liquid: 80 mg/15 mL, 10 mg/mL] q6-8h.
-Theo-Dur [100, 200, 300, 450 mg tabs; scored, may cut in half; do not crush]
q8-12h.
-Theophylline Products
Cap: 100, 200 mg
Cap, SR: 50, 60, 65, 75, 100, 125, 130, 200, 250, 260, 300 mg
Liquid: 80 mg/15 mL, 10 mg/mL
Tab: 100, 125, 200, 250, 300 mg
Tab, SR: 50, 75, 100, 125, 130, 200, 250, 260, 300, 400, 450, 500 mg

Corticosteroid metered dose inhalers or nebulized solution:
  -Beclomethasone (Beclovent, Vanceril) MDI 1-4 puffs bid-qid with spacer and mask, followed by gargling with water. [42 mcg/puff].
  -Beclomethasone (Vanceril Double Strength) MDI 2 puffs bid [84 mcg/puff]
  -Budesonide (Pulmicort Turbohaler) MDI 1-2 puffs bid [200 mcg/puff]
  -Budesonide (Pulmicort) 0.25-0.5 mg nebulized bid [0.25 mg/2mL, 0.5 mg/2mL]
  -Flunisolide (Aerobid) MDI 2-4 puffs bid [250 mcg/puff]
  -Fluticasone (Flovent) MDI 1-2 puffs bid [44, 110, 220 mcg/actuation]
  -Triamcinolone (Azmacort) MDI 1-4 puffs bid-qid [100 mcg/puff]
Cromolyn/nedocromil:
  -Cromolyn sodium (Intal) MDI 2-4 puffs qid [800 mcg/puff] or nebulized 20 mg bid-qid [10 mg/mL 2 mL unit dose ampules]
  -Nedocromil (Tilade) MDI 2 puffs bid-qid [1.75 mg/puff]
Oral beta-$_2$ agonists:
  -Albuterol (Proventil)
      2-6 years: 0.1-0.2 mg/kg/dose PO q6-8h
      6-12 years: 2 mg PO tid-qid
      >12 years: 2-4 mg PO tid-qid or 4-8 mg ER tab PO bid
      [soln: 2 mg/5 mL; tab: 2, 4 mg; tab, ER: 4, 8 mg]
  -Metaproterenol (Alupent, Metaprel)
      < 2 years: 0.4 mg/kg/dose PO tid-qid
      2-6 years: 1.3-2.6 mg PO q6-8h
      6-9 years: 10 mg PO q6-8h
      [syrup: 10 mg/5mL; tabs: 10, 20 mg]
Leukotriene receptor antagonists:
  -Montelukast (Singulair)
      2-5 year: 4 mg PO qPM
      6-14 year: 5 mg PO qPM
      > 14 year: 10 mg PO qPM
      [tab: 10 mg; tab, chew : 4, 5 mg]
  -Zafirlukast (Accolate)
      7-11 year: 10 mg PO bid
      $\geq$12 year: 20 mg PO bid
      [tabs: 10, 20 mg]
  -Zileuton (Zyflo)
      $\geq$12 year: 600 mg PO qid (with meals and at bedtime)
      [tab: 600 mg]
10. **Extras and X-rays:** CXR, pulmonary function test, peak flow rates.
11. **Labs:** CBC, CBG/ABG. Urine antigen screen, UA, theophylline level.

Allergic Rhinitis and Conjunctivitis

Antihistamines:
-Astemizole (Hismanal):
  6-12 year: 5 mg/day PO qd
  >12 year: 10 mg PO qd
  [tab: 10 mg].
-Loratadine (Claritin)
  >3 years and < 30 kg: 5 mg PO qd
  >30 kg: 10 mg PO qd.
  [syrup: 1mg/mL; tab: 10 mg; tab, rapidly disintegrating: 10 mg]
-Cetirizine (Zyrtec)
  12 year: 5-10 mg qd
  6-11 year: 5-10 mg qd
  [tabs: 5, 10 mg Syrup: 5 mg/5 mL]
-Fexofenadine (Allegra), 12 year: 60 mg bid [60 mg]
-Actifed [per cap or tab or 10 mL syrup: triprolidine 2.5 mg, pseudoephedrine
  60 mg]
  4 mg pseudoephedrine/kg/day PO tid-qid **OR**
  4 month-2 year: 1.25 mL PO q6-8h
  2-4 year: 2.5 mL PO q6-8h
  4-6 year: 3.75 mL PO q6-8h
  6-11y: 5 mL or 1/2 tab PO q6-8h
  >12 year: 10 mL or 1 cap/tab PO q6-8h.
-Chlorpheniramine maleate (Chlor-Trimeton):
  0.35 mg/kg/day PO q4-6h OR
  2-5 year: 1 mg PO q4-6h (max 4 mg/day)
  6-11year: 2 mg PO q4-6h (max 12 mg/day)
  >12year: 4 mg PO q4-6h or 8-12 mg SR q8-12h (max 24 mg/day).
  [cap, SR: 8,12 mg; soln: 2 mg/5 mL; tab: 4, 8, 12 mg; tab, chew: 2 mg;
  tab, SR: 8, 12 mg]
-Diphenhydramine (Benadryl)
  1 mg/kg/dose PO q6h prn, max 50 mg/dose
  [elixir/liquid: 12.5 mg/5 mL; tab, cap: 25, 50 mg].

Intranasal Therapy:
-Azelastine (Astelin)
  3-12 year: 1 spray in each nostril bid
  >12 year: 2 sprays in each nostril bid
  [nasal soln: 1 mg/mL, 17 mL (137 mcg/spray)]
-Beclomethasone (Beconase, Vancenase)
  6-11 years: 1 spray into each nostril tid
  >12 years: 1 spray into each nostril bid-qid
  [42 mcg/actuation]

-Beclomethasone aqueous (Beconase AQ)

   6-11 years: 1-2 sprays into each nostril bid

   $\geq$12 years: 1-2 sprays into each nostril bid

   [42 mcg/actuation]

-Beclomethasone Double Strength (Vancenase AQ)

   6-11 years: 1-2 puffs into each nostril qd

   $\geq$12 years: 1-2 sprays into each nostril qd

   [84 mcg/actuation]

-Budesonide (Rhinocort)

   6-11 years: 2 sprays into each nostril bid or 4 sprays into each nostril qAM

   $\geq$12 years: 2 sprays into each nostril bid or 4 sprays into each nostril qAM

   [32 mcg/actuation]

-Budesonide aqueous(Rhinocort AQ)

   6-11 years: 1-2 sprays into each nostril bid

   $\geq$12 years: 1 sprays into each nostril qd, may increase up to 4 sprays into each nostril qAM

   [32 mcg/actuation]

-Cromolyn (Nasalcrom)

   1 puff into each nostril q3-4h

   [40 mg/mL 13 mL].

-Flunisolide (Nasalide, Nasarel)

   6-11 years: 1 spray into each nostril tid or 2 sprays into each nostril bid

   $\geq$12 years: 2 sprays into each nostril bid-tid

   [25 mcg/actuation].

-Fluticasone (Flonase)

   4-6 years: 1-2 sprays into each nostril qd

   6-11 years: 1-2 sprays into each nostril qd

   $\geq$ 12 years: 1 spray into each nostril bid or 2 sprays into each nostril qd

   [50 mcg/actuation]

-Mometasone (Nasonex)

   4-6 years: 1 spray into each nostril qd

   6-11 years: 1 spray into each nostril qd

   $\geq$12 years: 2 sprays into each nostril qd

   [50 mcg/actuation]

-Triamcinolone (Nasacort)

   6-11 year: 2 sprays into each nostril qd

   >12 year: 2 sprays into each nostril qd.

   [55 mcg/actuation]

-Triamcinolone aqueous (Nasacort AQ)

   6-11 year: 2 spray into each nostril qd

   >12 year: 2 sprays into each nostril qd.

   [55 mcg/actuation]

Allergic Conjunctivitis Therapy:

-Azelastine (Optivar)

   $\geq$3 year: instill 1 drop into affected eye(s) bid

[ophth soln: 0.05% 6 mL]

-Cromolyn ophthalmic (Crolom, Opticrom)

Instill 2 drops into each affected eye(s) q4-6h

[ophth soln: 4% 2.5, 10 mL].

Decongestants:

-Pseudoephedrine (Sudafed, Novafed)

<12 year: 4 mg/kg/day PO q6h.

>12 year and adults: 30-60 mg/dose PO q6-8h or sustained release 120 mg PO q12h or sustained release 240 mg PO q24h

[cap/caplet, SR: 120, 240 mg; drops: 7.5 mg/0.8mL; syrup: 15 mg/5mL, 30 mg/5mL; tabs: 30, 60 mg]

Anaphylaxis

1. **Admit to:**
2. **Diagnosis:** Anaphylaxis.
3. **Condition:**
4. **Vital signs:** Call MD if:
5. **Activity:**
6. **Nursing:** Inputs and outputs, pulse oximeter.
7. **Diet:**
8. **IV Fluids:** 2 IV lines. Normal saline or LR 10-20 mL/kg rapidly over 1h, then D5 1/2 NS at 1-1.5 times maintenance.
9. **Special Medications:**

-O_2 at 4 L/min by NC or mask.

-Epinephrine, 0.01 mg/kg [0.01 mL/kg of 1 mg/mL = 1:1000] (maximum 0.5 mL) subcutaneously, repeat every 15-20 minutes prn. Usual dose for infants is 0.05-0.1mL, for children 0.1-0.3 mL, and for adolescents 0.3-0.5 mL. If anaphylaxis is caused by an insect sting or intramuscular injection, inject an additional 0.1 mL of epinephrine at the site to slow antigen absorption.

-Epinephrine racemic (if stridor is present), 2.25% nebulized, 0.25-0.5 mL in 2.5 mL NS over 15 min q30 min-4h.

-Albuterol (Ventolin [0.5%, 5 mg/mL soln]) nebulized 0.01-0.03 mL/kg (max 1 mL) in 2 mL NS q1-2h and prn; may be used in addition to epinephrine if necessary.

Corticosteroids:

-For severe symptoms, give hydrocortisone 5 mg/kg IV q8h until stable, then change to oral prednisone. If symptoms are mild, give prednisone: initially 2 mg/kg/day (max 40 mg) PO q12h, then taper the dose over 4-5 days.

Antihistamines:

-Diphenhydramine (Benadryl) 1 mg/kg/dose IV/IM/IO/PO q6h, max 50 mg/dose **OR**

-Hydroxyzine (Vistaril) 0.5-1 mg/kg/dose IM/IV/PO q4-6h, max 50 mg/dose.
10. **Extras and X-rays:** Portable CXR.
11. **Labs:** CBC, SMA 7, ABG.

Pleural Effusion

1. **Admit to:**
2. **Diagnosis:** Pleural effusion.
3. **Condition:**
4. **Vital signs:** Call MD if:
5. **Activity:**
6. **Diet:**
7. **IV Fluids:**
8. **Extras and X-rays:** CXR PA and LAT, lateral decubitus, ultrasound, sputum AFB. Pulmonary consult.
9. **Labs:** CBC with differential, SMA 7, protein, albumin, ESR, UA.

Pleural fluid:

> **Tube 1** - LDH, protein, amylase, triglycerides, glucose, specific gravity (10 mL red top).
>
> **Tube 2** - Gram stain, culture and sensitivity, AFB, fungal culture and sensitivity (20-60 mL).
>
> **Tube 3** - Cell count and differential (5-10 mL, EDTA purple top).
>
> **Tube 4** - Cytology (25-50 mL, heparinized).
>
> **Syringe** - pH (2 mL, heparinized).

Evaluation of Thoracentesis Fluid		
	Transudate	**Exudate**
Specific gravity	<1.016	>1.016
Protein ratio pleural fluid/serum	<0.5	>0.5
Protein (gm/100 mL)	<3.0	>3.0
LDH ratio pleural fluid/serum	<0.6	>0.6
WBC	<1,000/mm^3	>1,000/mm^3
Glucose	Equivalent to serum	Less than serum

Infectious Diseases

Suspected Sepsis

1. **Admit to:**
2. **Diagnosis:** Suspected sepsis.
3. **Condition:**
4. **Vital signs:** Call MD if:
5. **Activity:**
6. **Nursing:** Inputs and outputs, daily weights, cooling measures prn temp >38°C, consent for lumbar puncture.
7. **Diet:**
8. **IV Fluids:** Correct hypovolemia if present; NS 10-20 mL/kg IV bolus, then IV fluids at 1-1.5 times maintenance.
9. **Special medications:**

Term newborns <1 month old (Group B strep, E coli, Group D strep, gram negatives, Listeria monocytogenes): Ampicillin and gentamicin or cefotaxime.

-Ampicillin IV/IM: <7 days: 150 mg/kg/day q8h; >7 days: 200 mg/kg/day q6h **AND**

-Cefotaxime (Claforan) IV/IM: <7 days: 100 mg/kg/day q12h; >7 days: 150 mg/kg/day q8h **OR**

-Gentamicin (Garamycin) IV/IM: 5 mg/kg/day q12h.

-Also see page 117.

Infant 1-2 months old (H. flu, strep pneumonia, N meningitidis, Group B strep):

-Ampicillin 100 mg/kg/day IV/IM q6h **AND EITHER**

-Cefotaxime (Claforan) 100 mg/kg/day IV/IM q6h **OR**

-Ceftriaxone (Rocephin) 50-75 mg/kg/day IV/IM q12-24h **OR**

-Gentamicin (Garamycin) 7.5 mg/kg/day IV/IM q8h

Children 2 months to 18 years old (S pneumonia, H flu, N. meningitidis):

-Cefotaxime (Claforan) 100 mg/kg/day IV/IM q6h, max 12 gm/day **OR**

-Ceftriaxone (Rocephin) 50-75 mg/kg/day IV/IM q 12-24h, max 4 gm/day.

Immunocompromised Patients (Gram negative bacilli, Pseudomonas, Staph, Strep viridans):

-Ticarcillin (Ticar) 200-300 mg/kg/day IV/IM q6h, max 24 gm/day

-Ticarcillin/clavulanate (Timentin) 200-300 mg/kg/day of ticarcillin IV/IM q6-8h, max 24gm/day **OR**

-Piperacillin (Pipracil) 200-300 mg/kg/day IV/IM q6h, max 24 gm/day **OR**

-Piperacillin/Tazobactam (Zosyn) 240 mg/kg/day of piperacillin IV/IM q6-8h, max 12 gm/day **OR**

-Ceftazidime (Fortaz) 100-150 mg/kg/day IV/IM q8h, max 12 gm/day **AND**

-Tobramycin (Nebcin) or Gentamicin (Garamycin) (normal renal function):

   <5 year (except neonates): 7.5 mg/kg/day IV/IM q8h.

   5-10 year: 6.0 mg/kg/day IV/IM q8h.

   >10 year: 5.0 mg/kg/day IV/IM q8h **AND (if gram positive infection strongly suspected)**

-Vancomycin (Vancocin) (central line infection) 40-60 mg/kg/day IV q6-8h, max 4 gm/day

10. **Symptomatic medications:**

   -Ibuprofen (Advil) 5-10 mg/kg/dose PO q6h-8h prn temp >38°C **OR**

   -Acetaminophen (Tylenol) 10-15 mg/kg PO/PR q4-6h prn temp >38°C or pain.

11. **Extras and X-rays:** CXR.

12. **Labs:** CBC, SMA 7. Blood culture and sensitivity x 2. UA, urine culture; antibiotic levels. Stool for Wright stain if diarrhea. Nasopharyngeal washings for direct fluorescent antibody (RSV, chlamydia).

   CSF Tube 1 - Gram stain, culture and sensitivity for bacteria, antigen screen (1-2 mL).

   CSF Tube 2 - Glucose, protein (1-2 mL).

   CSF Tube 3 - Cell count and differential (1-2 mL).

Meningitis

1. **Admit to:**
2. **Diagnosis:** Meningitis.
3. **Condition:** Guarded.
4. **Vital signs:** Call MD if:
5. **Activity:**
6. **Nursing:** Strict isolation precautions. Inputs and outputs, daily weights; cooling measures prn temp >38°C; consent for lumbar puncture.
7. **Diet:**
8. **IV Fluids:** Isotonic fluids at maintenance rate.
9. **Special Medications:**

Term Newborns <1 months old (Group B strep, E coli, gram negatives, Listeria):

   -Ampicillin, 0-7 days: 150 mg/kg/day IV/IM q8h; >7days: 200 mg/kg/day IV/IM q6h **AND**

   -Cefotaxime (Claforan): <7days: 100 mg/kg/day IV/IM q12h; >7 days: 150 mg/kg/day q8h IV/IM.

Infants 1-3 months old (H. flu, strep pneumonia, N. Meningitidis, group B strep, E coli):

   -Cefotaxime (Claforan) 200 mg/kg/day IV/IM q6h **OR**

   -Ceftriaxone (Rocephin) 100 mg/kg/day IV/IM q12-24h **AND**

-Vancomycin (Vancocin) 40-60 mg/kg/day IV q6h.

-Dexamethasone 0.6 mg/kg/day IV q6h x 4 days. Initiate before or with the first dose of parenteral antibiotic.

Children 3 months to 18 years old (S pneumonia, H flu, N. meningitidis):

-Cefotaxime (Claforan) 200 mg/kg/day IV/IM q6h, max 12 gm/day or ceftriaxone (Rocephin) 100 mg/kg/day IV/IM q12-24h, max 4 gm/day **AND**

-Vancomycin (Vancocin) 60 mg/kg/day IV q6h, max 4gm/day.

-Dexamethasone 0.6 mg/kg/day IV q6h x 4 days. Initiate before or with the first dose of parenteral antibiotic.

10. **Symptomatic Medications:**

-Ibuprofen (Advil) 5-10 mg/kg/dose PO q6-8h prn **OR**

-Acetaminophen (Tylenol) 15 mg/kg PO/PR q4h prn temp >38°C or pain.

11. **Extras and X-rays:** CXR.

12. **Labs:** CBC, SMA 7. Blood culture and sensitivity x 2. UA, urine culture and sensitivity; urine specific gravity. Antibiotic levels. Urine and blood antigen testing.

Lumbar Puncture:

CSF Tube 1 - Gram stain, culture and sensitivity, bacterial antigen screen (1-2 mL).

CSF Tube 2 - Glucose, protein (1-2 mL).

CSF Tube 3 - Cell count and differential (1-2 mL).

Specific Therapy for Meningitis and Encephalitis

Dexamethasone (0.6 mg/kg/day IV q6h x 4 days) given before the first dose of antibiotics decreases hearing deficits in Haemophilus influenzae meningitis.

Streptococcus pneumoniae:

Until sensitivities are available, combination therapy with vancomycin and cefotaxime/ceftriaxone is recommended. For children with severe hypersensitivity to beta lactams, vancomycin and rifampin are recommended.

-Penicillin G 250,000-400,000 U/kg/day IV/IM q4-6h, max 24 MU/day

-Cefotaxime (Claforan) 200-300 mg/kg/day IV/IM q6h, max 12 gm/day

-Ceftriaxone (Rocephin) 100 mg/kg/day IV/IM q12-24h, max 4 gm/day

-Vancomycin (Vancocin) 60 mg/kg/day IV q6h, max 4 gm/day

-Rifampin 20 mg/kg/day IV q12h, max 600 mg/day

-Meropenem (Merrem) 120 mg/kg/day IV q8h, max 6 gm/day

-Chloramphenicol (Chloromycetin) 75-100 mg/kg/day IV q6h, max 4 gm/day

Neisseria meningitidis:

Penicillin is the drug of choice. Cefotaxime and ceftriaxone are acceptable alternatives.

-Penicillin G 250,000-400,000 U/kg/day IV/IM q4h x 7-10d, max 24 MU/d.

-Cefotaxime (Claforan) 200-300 mg/kg/day IV/IM q6h, max 12 gm/day

-Ceftriaxone (Rocephin) 100 mg/kg/day IV/IM q12-24h, max 4 gm/day

Meningococcal exposure prophylaxis (see H flu prophylaxis below):

-Ceftriaxone (Rocephin) IM x 1 dose; $\leq$12year: 125 mg; >12year: 250 mg **OR**

-Rifampin, $\leq$1month: 5 mg/kg/dose PO bid x 2 days; >1 month: 10 mg/kg/dose (max 600 mg/dose) PO q12h x 2 days [caps: 150 mg, 300 mg; suspension] **OR**

-Ciprofloxacin (Cipro) 500 mg PO x 1 for adults (>18 year).

Haemophilus influenzae

Ampicillin should not be used alone as initial therapy until sensitivities are available because 10-40% of isolates are ampicillin-resistant.

-Cefotaxime (Claforan) 200-300 mg/kg/day IV/IM q6h, max 12 gm/day **OR**

-Ceftriaxone (Rocephin) 100 mg/kg/day IV/IM q12-24h, max 4 gm/day **OR**

-Ampicillin (beta-lactamase negative) 200-400 mg/kg/day IV/IM q4-6h, max 12 gm/day.

H influenzae type B exposure prophylaxis and eradication of nasopharyngeal carriage:

-Rifampin <1 month: 10 mg/kg/day PO q24h x 4 days; >1 month: 20 mg/kg/day PO qd x 4 doses (max 600 mg/dose). [caps: 150, 300 mg; suspension].

Group A or non-enterococcal Group D Streptococcus:

-Penicillin G 250,000 U/kg/day IV/IM q4-6h, max 24 MU/d.

Listeria monocytogenes or Group B Streptococcus:

-Ampicillin 200 mg/kg/day IV/IM q6h, max 12 gm/day **AND**

-Gentamicin (Garamycin) or Tobramycin (Nebcin) (normal renal function):

<5 year (except neonates): 7.5 mg/kg/day IV/IM q8h.

5-10 year: 6.0 mg/kg/day IV/IM q8h.

>10 year: 5.0 mg/kg/day IV/IM q8h

Staphylococcus aureus:

-Nafcillin (Nafcil) or Oxacillin (Bactocill, Prostaphlin)150-200 mg/kg/day IV/IM q4-6h, max 12 gm/day **OR**

-Vancomycin (Vancocin) 40-60 mg/kg/day IV q6h, max 4 gm/day (may require concomitant intrathecal therapy).

Herpes Simplex Encephalitis:

-Acyclovir (Zovirax) 1500 mg/m^2/day or 30 mg/kg/day IV over 1h q8h x 14-21 days

Infective Endocarditis

1. **Admit to:**
2. **Diagnosis:** Infective endocarditis.
3. **Condition:**
4. **Vital signs:** Call MD if:
5. **Activity:**
6. **Diet:**
7. **IV Fluids:**
8. **Special Medications:**

Subacute Bacterial Endocarditis Empiric Therapy:
   - Penicillin G 250,000 U/kg/day IV/IM q4-6, max 24 MU/day **AND**
   - Gentamicin (Garamycin) or Tobramycin (Nebcin) (normal renal function):
     <5 year (except neonates): 7.5 mg/kg/day IV/IM q8h.
     5-10 year: 6.0 mg/kg/day IV/IM q8h.
     >10 year: 5.0 mg/kg/day IV/IM q8h

Acute Bacterial Endocarditis Empiric Therapy (including IV drug user):
   - Gentamicin (Garamycin) or Tobramycin (Nebcin), see above for dose **AND EITHER**
   - Nafcillin (Nafcil) or oxacillin (Bactocill, Prostaphlin) 150 mg/kg/day IV/IM q6h, max 12 gm/day **OR**
   - Vancomycin (Vancocin) 40-60 mg/kg/day IV q6-8h, max 4 gm/day

Streptococci viridans/bovis:
   - Penicillin G 150,000 u/kg/day IV/IM q4-6h, max 24 MU/day **OR**
   - Vancomycin (Vancocin) 40-60 mg/kg/day IV q6-8h, max 4 gm/day.

Staphylococcus aureus (methicillin sensitive):
   - Nafcillin (Nafcil) or oxacillin (Bactocill, Prostaphlin) 150 mg/kg/day IV/IM q6h, max 12 gm/day **AND**
   - Gentamicin (Garamycin) or Tobramycin (Nebcin), see dose above.

Methicillin-resistant Staphylococcus aureus:
   - Vancomycin (Vancocin) 40-60 mg/kg/day IV q6h, max 4 gm/day.

Staphylococcus epidermidis:
   - Vancomycin (Vancocin) 40-60 mg/kg/day IV q6h max 4 gm/day **AND**
   - Gentamicin (Garamycin) or Tobramycin (Nebcin), see dose above.

9. **Extras and X-rays:** CXR PA and LAT, echocardiogram, ECG. Cardiology and infectious disease consultation.
10. **Labs:** CBC, ESR. Bacterial culture and sensitivity x 3-4 over 24h, MBC. Antibiotic levels. UA, urine culture and sensitivity.

Endocarditis Prophylaxis

Prophylactic Regimens for Dental, Oral, Respiratory Tract, or Esophageal Procedures			
Situation	**Drug**	**Regimen**	**Maximum Dose**
Standard general prophylaxis	Amoxicillin	50 mg/kg PO as a single dose 1 hr before procedure	2000 mg
Unable to take oral medication	Ampicillin	50 mg/kg IV/IM within 30 minutes before procedure	2000 mg
Allergic to penicillin	Clindamycin **or**	20 mg/kg PO as a single dose 1 hour before procedure	600 mg
	Cephalexin (Keflex) or cefadroxil (Duricef) **or**	50 mg/kg PO as a single dose 1 hour before procedure	2000 mg
	Azithromycin (Zithromax) or clarithromycin (Biaxin)	15 mg/kg PO as a single dose 1 hour before procedure	500 mg
Allergic to penicillin and unable to take oral medications	Clindamycin **or**	20 mg/kg IV 30 minutes before procedure	600 mg
	Cefazolin (Ancef)	25 mg/kg IV/IM within 30 minutes before procedure	1000 mg

Prophylactic Regimens for Genitourinary/Gastrointestinal Procedures			
Situation	**Drug**	**Regimen**	**Maximum Dose**
High-risk patients	Ampicillin **plus**	50 mg/kg IV/IM	2000 mg
	Gentamicin followed by	1.5 mg/kg IV/IM within 30 minutes before starting procedure	120 mg
	Ampicillin or Amoxicillin	25 mg/kg IV/IM 25 mg/kg PO six hours later	1000 mg 1000 mg

Situation	Drug	Regimen	Maximum Dose
High-risk patients allergic to penicillin	Vancomycin **plus**	20 mg/kg IV over 1-2 hours	1000 mg
	Gentamicin	1.5 mg/kg IV/IM to be completed within 30 minutes before starting procedure	120 mg
Moderate-risk Patients	Amoxicillin **or**	50 mg/kg PO one hour before procedure	2000 mg
	Ampicillin	50 mg/kg IV/IM within 30 minutes of starting pro-cedure	2000 mg
Moderate-risk patients allergic to penicillin	Vancomycin	20 mg/kg IV over 1-2 hours, completed within 30 minutes of starting the procedure	1000 mg

Pneumonia

1. **Admit to:**
2. **Diagnosis:** Pneumonia.
3. **Condition:**
4. **Vital signs:** Call MD if:
5. **Activity:**
6. **Nursing:** Pulse oximeter, inputs and outputs. Bronchial clearance techniques, vibrating vest.
7. **Diet:**
8. **IV Fluids:**
9. **Special Medications:**
   -Humidified O_2 by NC at 2-4 L/min or 25-100% by mask, adjust to keep saturation >92%

Term Neonates <1 month:
   -Ampicillin 100 mg/kg/day IV/IM q6h **AND**
   -Cefotaxime (Claforan) <1 week: 100 mg/kg/day IV/IM q12h; >1 week: 150 mg/kg/day IV/IM q8h **OR**
   -Gentamicin (Garamycin) 5 mg/kg/day IV/IM q12h.

Children 1 month-5 years old:
   -Cefuroxime (Zinacef) 100-150 mg/kg/day IV/IM q8h **OR**

-Ampicillin 100 mg/kg/day IV/IM q6h **AND**

-Gentamicin (Garamycin) or Tobramycin (Nebcin):

    7.5 mg/kg/day IV/IM q8h (normal renal function).

-If chlamydia is strongly suspected, add erythromycin 40 mg/kg/day IV q6h.

Oral Therapy:

-Cefuroxime axetil (Ceftin)

    tab: child: 125-250 mg PO bid; adult: 250-500 mg PO bid

    susp: 30 mg/kg/day PO q12h, max 1000 mg/day

    [susp: 125 mg/5 mL; tabs: 125, 250,500 mg] **OR**

-Loracarbef (Lorabid)

    30 mg/kg/day PO q12h, max 800 mg/day

    [cap: 200, 400 mg; susp: 100 mg/5 mL, 200 mg/5mL]

-Cefpodoxime (Vantin)

    10 mg/kg/day PO q12h, max 800 mg/day

    [susp: 50 mg/5 mL, 100 mg/5 mL; tabs: 100, 200 mg]

-Cefprozil (Cefzil)

    30 mg/kg/day PO q12h, max 1000 mg/day

    [susp: 125 mg/5 mL, 250 mg/5 mL; tabs: 250, 500 mg].

-Cefixime (Suprax)

    8 mg/kg/day PO qd-bid, max 400 mg/day

    [susp: 100 mg/5 mL; tabs: 200, 400 mg].

-Clarithromycin (Biaxin)

    15-30 mg/kg/day PO bid, max 1000 mg/day

    [susp: 125 mg/5 mL, 250 mg/5 mL; tabs: 250, 500 mg].

-Azithromycin (Zithromax)

    Children $\geq$2 years: 12 mg/kg/day PO qd x 5 days, max 500 mg/day

    $\geq$16 years: 500 mg PO on day 1, 250 mg PO qd on days 2-5

    [cap: 250 mg; susp: 100 mg/5mL, 200 mg/5mL; tabs: 250, 600 mg]

-Amoxicillin/clavulanate (Augmentin)

    30-40 mg/kg/day of amoxicillin PO q8h , max 500 mg/dose

    [elixir 125 mg/5 mL, 250 mg/5 mL; tabs: 250, 500 mg; tabs, chew: 125, 250 mg;]

-Amoxicillin/clavulanate (Augmentin BID)

    30-40 mg/kg/day PO q12h, max 875 mg (amoxicillin)/dose

    [susp 200 mg/5 mL, 400 mg/5 mL; tab: 875 mg; tabs, chew: 200, 400 mg]

Community-Acquired Pneumonia 5-18 years old (viral, Mycoplasma pneumoniae, chlamydia pneumoniae, pneumococcus, legionella):

-Cefuroxime (Zinacef) 100-150 mg/kg/day IV/IM q8h, max 9 gm/day **OR**

-Erythromycin estolate (Ilosone) 30-50 mg/kg/day PO q8-12h, max 2 gm/day

    [caps: 125, 250 mg; drops: 100 mg/mL; susp: 125 mg/5 mL, 250 mg/5 mL; tab: 500 mg; tabs, chew: 125,250 mg]

-Erythromycin ethylsuccinate (EryPed, EES)

    30-50 mg/kg/day PO q6-8h, max 2gm/day

    [susp: 200 mg/5 mL, 400 mg/5 mL; tab: 400 mg; tab, chew: 200 mg]

-Erythromycin base (E-mycin, Ery-Tab, Eryc)
   30-50 mg/kg/day PO q6-8h, max 2gm/day
   [cap, DR: 250 mg; tabs: 250, 333, 500 mg]
-Erythromycin lactobionate
   20-40 mg/kg/day IV q6h, max 4 gm/day
   [inj: 500 mg, 1 gm]
-Clarithromycin (Biaxin)
   15-30 mg/kg/day PO bid, max 1000 mg/day
   [susp: 125 mg/5 mL, 250 mg/5 mL; tabs: 250, 500 mg]

Immunosuppressed, Neutropenic Pneumonia (S. pneumoniae, group A strep, H flu, gram neg enterics, Klebsiella, Mycoplasma Pneumonia, Legionella, Chlamydia pneumoniae, S aureus):

-Tobramycin (Nebcin) (normal renal function):
   <5 year (except neonates): 7.5 mg/kg/day IV/IM q8h.
   5-10 year: 6.0 mg/kg/day IV/IM q8h.
   >10 year: 5.0 mg/kg/day IV/IM q8h **OR**
-Ceftazidime (Fortaz) 150 mg/kg/day IV/IM q8h, max 12 gm/day **AND**
-Ticarcillin/Clavulanate (Timentin) 200-300 mg/kg/day of ticarcillin IV q6-8h,
   max 24 gm/day **OR**
-Nafcillin (Nafcil) or oxacillin (Bactocill, Prostaphlin) 150 mg/kg/day IV/IM q6h,
   max 12 gm/day **OR**
-Vancomycin (Vancocin) 40 mg/kg/day IV q6h, max 4 gm/day.

Cystic Fibrosis Exacerbation (Pseudomonas aeruginosa):

-Ticarcillin/clavulanate (Timentin) 200-300 mg/kg/day of ticarcillin IV q6-8h,
   max 24 gm/day **OR**
-Piperacillin/tazobactam (Zosyn) 300 mg/kg/day of piperacillin IV q6-8h, max
   12 gm/day **OR**
-Piperacillin (Pipracil) 200-300 mg/kg/day IV/IM q4-6h, max 24 gm/day **AND**
-Tobramycin (Nebcin):
   <5 year (except neonates): 7.5 mg/kg/day IV/IM q8h.
   5-10 year: 6.0 mg/kg/day IV/IM q8h.
   >10 year: 5.0 mg/kg/day IV/IM q8h **OR**
-Ceftazidime (Fortaz) 150 mg/kg/day IV/IM q8h, max 12 gm/day **OR**
-Aztreonam (Azactam) 150-200 mg/kg/day IV/IM q6-8h, max 8 gm/day **OR**
-Imipenem/cilastatin (Primaxin) 60-100 mg/kg/day of imipenem IV q6-8h, max
   4 gm/day **OR**
-Meropenem (Merrem) 60-120 mg/kg/day IV q8h, max 6gm/day.

10. **Symptomatic Medications:**
   -Acetaminophen (Tylenol) 10-15 mg/kg PO/PR q4h prn temp >38°C or pain.
11. **Extras and X-rays:** CXR PA and LAT, PPD
12. **Labs:** CBC, ABG, blood culture and sensitivity x 2. Sputum gram stain, culture and sensitivity, AFB. Antibiotic levels. Nasopharyngeal washings for direct fluorescent antibody (RSV, adenovirus, parainfluenza, influenza virus, chlamydia) and cultures for respiratory viruses. UA.

Specific Therapy for Pneumonia

Pneumococcal pneumonia:
  -Erythromycin estolate (Ilosone)
    30-50 mg/kg/day PO q8-12h, max 2 gm/day
    [caps: 125, 250 mg; drops: 100 mg/mL; susp: 125 mg/5 mL, 250 mg/5 mL;
    tab: 500 mg; tabs, chew: 125,250 mg]
  -Erythromycin ethylsuccinate (EryPed, EES)
    30-50 mg/kg/day PO q6-8h, max 2gm/day
    [susp: 200 mg/5 mL, 400 mg/5 mL; tab: 400 mg; tab, chew: 200 mg]
  -Erythromycin base (E-Mycin, Ery-Tab, Eryc)
    30-50 mg/kg/day PO q6-8h, max 2gm/day
    [tab: 250, 333, 500 mg]
  -Erythromycin lactobionate
    20-40 mg/kg/day IV q6h, max 4 gm/day
    [inj: 500 mg, 1 g m] **OR**
-Vancomycin (Vancocin) 40 mg/kg/day IV q6h, max 4 gm/day **OR**
-Cefotaxime (Claforan) 100-150 mg/kg/day IV/IM q6h, max 12 gm/day **OR**
-Penicillin G 150,000 U/kg/day IV/IM q4-6h, max 24 MU/day.

Staphylococcus aureus:
  -Oxacillin (Bactocill, Prostaphlin) or nafcillin (Nafcil) 150-200 mg/kg/day IV/IM
    q4-6h, max 12 gm/day **OR**
  -Vancomycin (Vancocin) 40 mg/kg/day IV q6h, max 4 gm/day

Haemophilus influenzae (<5 year of age):
  -Cefotaxime (Claforan) 100-150 mg/kg/day IV/IM q8h, max 12 gm/day **OR**
  -Cefuroxime (Zinacef) 100-150 mg/kg/day IV/IM q8h (beta-lactamase pos),
    max 9 gm/day **OR**
  -Ampicillin 100-200 mg/kg/day IV/IM q6h (beta-lactamase negative), max 12
    gm/day

Pseudomonas aeruginosa:
  -Tobramycin (Nebcin):
    <5 year (except neonates): 7.5 mg/kg/day IV/IM q8h.
    5-10 year: 6.0 mg/kg/day IV/IM q8h.
    >10 year: 5.0 mg/kg/day IV/IM q8h **AND**
  -Piperacillin (Pipracil) or ticarcillin (Ticar) 200-300 mg/kg/day IV/IM q4-6h,
    max 24 gm/day **OR**
  -Ceftazidime (Fortaz) 150 mg/kg/day IV/IM q8h, max 12 gm/day.

Mycoplasma pneumoniae:
  -Clarithromycin (Biaxin) 15-30 mg/kg/day PO q12h, max 1 gm/day
    [susp: 125 mg/5 mL, 250 mg/5 mL; tabs: 250, 500 mg].
  -Erythromycin estolate (Ilosone)
    30-50 mg/kg/day PO q8-12h, max 2 gm/day.
    [caps: 125, 250 mg; drops: 100 mg/mL; susp: 125 mg/5 mL, 250 mg/5 mL;

tab: 500 mg; tabs, chew: 125,250 mg].
-Erythromycin ethylsuccinate (EryPed, EES)
   30-50 mg/kg/day PO q6-8h, max 2gm/day.
   [susp: 200 mg/5 mL, 400 mg/5 mL; tab: 400 mg; tab, chew: 200 mg].
-Erythromycin base (E-Mycin, Ery-Tab, Eryc)
   30-50 mg/kg/day PO q6-8h, max 2gm/day.
   [cap, DR: 250 mg; tabs: 250, 333, 500 mg].
-Erythromycin lactobionate (Erythrocin)
   20-40 mg/kg/day IV q6h, max 4 gm/day.
   [inj: 500 mg, 1 gm].

Moraxella catarrhalis:

-Clarithromycin (Biaxin)
   15 mg/kg/day PO q12h, max 1 gm/day
   [susp: 125 mg/5 mL, 250 mg/5 mL; tabs: 250, 500 mg] **OR**
-Cefuroxime (Zinacef) 100-150 mg/kg/day IV/IM q8h, max 9 gm/day **OR**
-Erythromycin estolate (Ilosone)
   30-50 mg/kg/day PO q8-12h, max 2 gm/day
   [caps: 125, 250 mg; drops: 100 mg/mL; susp: 125 mg/5 mL, 250 mg/5 mL;
   tab: 500 mg; tabs, chew: 125,250 mg]
-Erythromycin ethylsuccinate (EryPed, EES)
   30-50 mg/kg/day PO q6-8h, max 2gm/day
   [susp: 200 mg/5 mL, 400 mg/5 mL; tab: 400 mg; tab, chew: 200 mg]
-Erythromycin base (E-Mycin, Ery-Tab, Eryc)
   30-50 mg/kg/day PO q6-8h, max 2gm/day
   [cap, DR: 250 mg; tabs: 250, 333, 500 mg]
-Erythromycin lactobionate (Erythrocin)
   20-40 mg/kg/day IV q6h, max 4 gm/day
   [inj: 500 mg, 1 gm] **OR**
-Trimethoprim/sulfamethoxazole (Bactrim, Septra)
   6-12 mg TMP/kg/day PO/IV q12h, max 320 mg TMP/day
   [inj per mL: TMP 16 mg/SMX 80 mg; susp per 5 mL: TMP 40 mg/SMX 200
   mg; tab DS: TMP 160 mg/SMX 800 mg; tab SS: TMP 80mg/SMX 400 mg]

Chlamydia pneumoniae (TWAR), psittaci, trachomatous:
-Erythromycin estolate (Ilosone)
   30-50 mg/kg/day PO q8-12h, max 2 gm/day
   [caps: 125, 250 mg; drops: 100 mg/mL; susp: 125 mg/5 mL, 250 mg/5 mL; tab: 500 mg; tabs, chew: 125,250 mg]
-Erythromycin ethylsuccinate (EryPed, EES)
   30-50 mg/kg/day PO q6-8h, max 2gm/day
   [susp: 200 mg/5 mL, 400 mg/5 mL; tab: 400 mg; tab, chew: 200 mg]
-Erythromycin base (E-Mycin, Ery-Tab, Eryc)
   30-50 mg/kg/day PO q6-8h, max 2gm/day
   [cap, DR: 250 mg; tabs: 250, 333, 500 mg]
-Erythromycin lactobionate (Erythrocin)
   20-40 mg/kg/day IV q6h, max 4 gm/day
   [inj: 500 mg, 1 gm] **OR**
-Azithromycin (Zithromax)
   children $\geq$2 years: 12 mg/kg/day PO qd x 5 days, max 500 mg/day
   $\geq$16 years: 500 mg PO on day one, then 250 mg PO qd on days 2-5
   [cap: 250 mg; susp: 100 mg/5mL, 200 mg/5mL; tabs: 250, 600 mg]

Influenza Virus:
-Oseltamivir (Tamiflu)
   $\geq$1 year and <15 kg: 30 mg PO bid
   15-23 kg: 45 mg PO bid
   >23 - 40 kg: 60 mg PO bid
   >40 kg: 75 mg PO bid
   >18 year: 75 mg PO bid
   [cap: 75 mg; susp: 12 mg/mL]
   Approved for treatment of uncomplicated influenza A or B when patient has been symptomatic no longer than 48 hrs **OR**
-Rimantadine (Flumadine)
   <10 year: 5 mg/kg/day PO qd, max 150 mg/day
   >10 year: 100 mg PO bid
   [syrup: 50 mg/5 mL; tab: 100 mg].
   Approved for treatment or prophylaxis of Influenza A. Not effective against Influenza B. **OR**
-Amantadine (Symmetrel)
   1-9 year: 5 mg/kg/day PO qd-bid, max 150 mg/day
   >9 year: 5 mg/kg/day PO qd-bid, max 200 mg/day
   [cap: 100 mg; syrup: 50 mg/5 mL].
   Approved for treatment or prophylaxis of Influenza A. Not effective against Influenza B.

Bronchiolitis

1. **Admit to:**
2. **Diagnosis:** Bronchiolitis.
3. **Condition:**
4. **Vital signs:** Call MD if:
5. **Activity:**
6. **Nursing:** Pulse oximeter, peak flow rate. Respiratory isolation.
7. **Diet:**
8. **IV Fluids:**
9. **Special Medications:**
   -Oxygen, humidified 1-4 L/min by NC or 40-60% by mask, keep sat >92%.

Nebulized Beta-$_2$ agonists:
   -Albuterol (Ventolin, Proventil) (5 mg/mL soln) nebulized 0.2-0.5 mL in 2 mL NS (0.10-0.15 mg/kg) q1-4h prn.

Treatment of Respiratory Syncytial Virus (severe lung disease or underlying cardiopulmonary disease):
   -Ribavirin (Virazole) therapy should be considered in high risk children <2 years with chronic lung disease or with history of premature birth less than 35 weeks gestational age. Ribavirin is administered as a 6 gm vial, aerosolized by SPAG nebulizer over 18-20h qd x 3-5 days, or 2 gm over 2 hrs q8h x 3-5 days.

Prophylaxis Against Respiratory Syncytial Virus:
   -Recommended use in high risk children <2 years with BPD who required medical management within the past six months, or with history of premature birth less than or equal to 28 weeks gestational age who are less than one year of age at start of RSV season, or with history of premature birth 29-32 weeks gestational age who are less than six months of age at start of RSV season.
   -Palivizumab (Synagis) 15 mg/kg IM once a month throughout RSV season (October-March)
   -RSV-IVIG (RespiGam) 750 mg/kg IV once a month throughout RSV season (October to March).

Influenza A:
   -Oseltamivir (Tamiflu)
      $\geq$1 year and <15 kg: 30 mg PO bid
      15-23 kg: 45 mg PO bid
      >23 - 40 kg: 60 mg PO bid
      >40 kg: 75 mg PO bid
      >18 year: 75 mg PO bid
      [cap: 75 mg; susp: 12 mg/mL]
      Approved for treatment of uncomplicated influenza A or B when patient has been symptomatic no longer than 48 hrs. **OR**

-Rimantadine (Flumadine)

    <10 year: 5 mg/kg/day PO qd, max 150 mg/day

    >10 year: 100 mg PO bid

    [syrup: 50 mg/5 mL; tab: 100 mg].

    Approved for treatment or prophylaxis of Influenza A. Not effective against Influenza B **OR**

-Amantadine (Symmetrel)

    1-9 year: 5 mg/kg/day PO qd-bid, max 150 mg/day

    >9 year: 5 mg/kg/day PO qd-bid, max 200 mg/day

    [cap: 100 mg; syrup: 50 mg/5 mL].

    Approved for treatment or prophylaxis of Influenza A. Not effective against Influenza B.

Pertussis:

The estolate salt is preferred because of greater penetration.

-Erythromycin estolate 50 mg/kg/day PO q8-12h, max 2 gm/day

    [caps: 125, 250 mg; drops: 100 mg/mL; susp: 125 mg/5 mL, 250 mg/5 mL; tab: 500 mg; tabs, chew: 125,250 mg]

-Erythromycin lactobionate (Erythrocin) 20-40 mg/kg/day IV q6h, max 4 gm/day

    [inj: 500 mg, 1 gm].

Oral Beta-$_2$ agonists and Acetaminophen:

-Albuterol liquid (Proventil, Ventolin)

    2-6 years: 0.1-0. mg/kg/dose PO q6-8h

    6-12 years: 2 mg PO tid-qid

    >12 years: 2-4 mg PO tid-qid

    [soln: 2 mg/5 mL; tabs: 2,4 mg; tabs, SR: 4, 8 mg]

-Acetaminophen (Tylenol) 10-15 mg/kg PO/PR q4-6h prn temp >38°.

10. **Extras and X-rays:** CXR.

11. **Labs:** CBC, SMA 7, CBG/ABG, UA. Urine antigen screen. Nasopharyngeal washings for direct fluorescent antibody (RSV, adenovirus, parainfluenza, influenza virus, chlamydia), viral culture.

Viral Laryngotracheitis (Croup)

1. **Admit to:**
2. **Diagnosis:** Croup.
3. **Condition:**
4. **Vital signs:** Call MD if:
5. **Activity:**
6. **Nursing:** Pulse oximeter, laryngoscope and endotracheal tube at bedside. Respiratory isolation, inputs and outputs.
7. **Diet:**
8. **IV Fluids:**

9. **Special Medications:**
  -Oxygen, cool mist, 1-2 L/min by NC or 40-60% by mask, keep sat >92%.
  -Racemic epinephrine (2.25% soln) 0.05 mL/kg/dose (max 0.5 mL) in 2-3 mL saline nebulized q1-6h.
  -Dexamethasone (Decadron) 0.25-0.5 mg/kg/dose IM/IV q6h prn, max dose 10 mg **OR**
  -Prednisone 1-2 mg/kg/day PO q12-24h x 3-5 days [syrup: 1mg/mL, 5 mg/mL; tabs: 1, 2.5, 5, 10, 20, 50 mg]
  -Prednisolone 1-2 mg/kg/day PO q12-24h x 3-5 days [5 mg/5 mL, Orapred 20.2mg/5mL, Prelone 15 mg/5 mL].

10. **Extras and X-rays:** CXR PA and LAT, posteroanterior X-ray of neck.
11. **Labs:** CBC, CBG/ABG, blood culture and sensitivity; UA, culture and sensitivity. Urine antigen screen.

Varicella Zoster Infections

Immunocompetent Patient
  A. Therapy with oral acyclovir is not recommended routinely for the treatment of uncomplicated varicella in the otherwise healthy child <12 years of age.
  B. Oral acyclovir may be given within 24 hours of the onset of rash. Administration results in a modest decrease in the duration and magnitude of fever and a decrease in the number and duration of skin lesions.
  C. Acyclovir (Zovirax) 80 mg/kg/day PO q6h for five days, max 3200 mg/day [cap: 200 mg; susp: 200 mg/5 mL; tabs: 400, 800 mg]

Immunocompromised Patient
  A. Intravenous acyclovir should be initiated early in the course of the illness. Therapy within 24 hours of rash onset maximizes efficacy. Oral acyclovir should not be used because of unreliable bioavailability.
  Dose: 500 mg/m^2/dose IV q8h x 7-10 days
  B. Varicella zoster immune globulin (VZIG) may be given shortly after exposure to prevent or modify the course of the disease. It is not effective once disease is established.
  Dose: 125 U per 10 kg body weight, IM, round up to nearest vial size to max of 625 U [vial: 125 U/1.25ml].

Ventriculoperitoneal Shunt Infection

1. **Admit to:**
2. **Diagnosis:** VP Shunt Infection.
3. **Condition:** Guarded.
4. **Vital signs:** Call MD if:
5. **Activity:**
6. **Nursing:** Inputs and outputs, daily weights; cooling measures prn temp >38°C.
7. **Diet:**
8. **IV Fluids:** Isotonic fluids at maintenance rate.
9. **Special Medications:**
   -Vancomycin 40-60 mg/kg/day IV q6-8h, max 4 gm/day **OR**
   -Nafcillin (Nafcil) or oxacillin (Bactocill, Prostaphlin) 150-200 mg/kg/day IV/IM q6h, max 12 gm/day.
10. **Symptomatic Medications:**
    -Ibuprofen 5-10 mg/kg/dose PO q6-8h prn **OR**
    -Acetaminophen 15 mg/kg PO/PR q4h prn temp >38°C or pain.
11. **Extras and X-rays:** Neurosurgery consultation. MRI.
12. **Labs:** CBC, SMA 7. Blood culture and sensitivity. CSF cell count, culture, sensitivity, Gram stain, CSF glucose, protein.

Pneumocystis Carinii Pneumonia

1. **Admit to:**
2. **Diagnosis:** Pneumocystis carinii pneumonia.
3. **Condition:**
4. **Vital signs:** Call MD if:
5. **Activity:**
6. **Nursing:** Daily weights.
7. **Diet:**
8. **Fluids:**
9. **Special Medications:**

Pneumocystis Carinii Pneumonia (PCP) Treatment:
   -Oxygen prn for hypoxia.
   -Trimethoprim/sulfamethoxazole (Bactrim, Septra) 15-20 mg TMP/kg/day IV/PO q6h x 14-21 days [inj per mL: TMP 16 mg/SMX 80 mg; susp per 5 mL: TMP 40 mg/SMX 200 mg; tab DS: TMP 160 mg/SMX 800 mg; tab SS: TMP 80mg/SMX 400 mg] x 14-21 days
   Oral therapy is reserved for patients with mild disease who do not have malabsorption or diarrhea **OR**
   -Pentamidine (Pentam) 4 mg/kg/day IV over 1-2h for 14-21days

-Prednisone:

> <13 years: 2mg/kg/day PO qd x 7-10 days, then taper over the next 10-14 days.

> >13 years old with hypoxia: 40 mg PO bid x 5 days, then 40 mg PO qd x 5 days, then 20 mg PO qd x 11 days.

Pneumocystis Carinii Pneumonia Prophylaxis:

-Trimethoprim/sulfamethoxazole (Bactrim, Septra) 150 mg/m^2 trimethoprim/kg/day PO bid three days per week. [inj per mL: TMP 16 mg/SMX 80 mg; susp per 5 mL: TMP 40 mg/SMX 200 mg; tab DS: TMP 160 mg/SMX 800 mg; tab SS: TMP 80/SMX 400 mg] **OR**

-Dapsone (Avlosulfon) ($\geq$1 mo) 2 mg/kg/day PO q24h, max 100 mg/day or 4 mg/kg/dose PO q week, max 200 mg/dose [tabs: 25,100 mg] **OR**

-Aerosolized Pentamidine (NebuPent) (if $\geq$5 years): 300 mg nebulized monthly

-Atovaquone (Mepron)

> 1-3 months and >24 months: 45 mg/kg/day PO qd

> 4-24 months: 30 mg/kg/day PO qd

> [liquid: 750 mg/5mL]

10. **Extras and X-rays:** CXR PA and LAT, PPD.

11. **Labs:** CBC, SMA 7, LDH. Blood culture and sensitivity x 2. Sputum Gram stain, culture and sensitivity. Sputum stain for Pneumocystis, AFB. CD4 count, HIV RNA PCR, UA.

AIDS

Antiretroviral Therapy:

-Zidovudine (Retrovir, AZT) - oral

> <2 weeks: 8 mg/kg/day PO q6h.

> 2-4 weeks: 12 mg/kg/day PO q6h.

> 4 wks -12 year: 90-180 mg/m^2/dose q6h, max 200 mg/dose.

> >12 year, monotherapy and asymptomatic: 100 mg q4h while awake (max 500 mg/day).

> >12 year, monotherapy and symptomatic: 100 mg q4h.

> >12 years and combination therapy: 200 mg PO q8h.

> [cap: 100 mg; soln: 10 mg/mL; tab: 300 mg].

-Zidovudine - intravenous

> <2 weeks: 6 mg/kg/day IV q6h.

> 2-4 weeks: 9 mg/kg/day IV q6h.

> 4 wks to 12 year: 0.5-1.8 mg/kg/hr continuous IV infusion or 100-120 mg/m^2/dose IV q6h.

> >12 year: 1 mg/kg/dose q4h.

> [inj: 10 mg/mL].

-Lamivudine (Epivir, 3TC)

      3 mos-12 year: 2-4 mg/kg/dose PO bid (max 150 mg/dose).

      >12 year: if <50kg: 2 mg/kg/dose PO bid; if $\geq$50kg: 150 mg PO bid.

      [soln: 10 mg/mL; tab: 150 mg].

-Didanosine (Videx, ddI)

      <90 days: 100 mg/m^2/day PO q12h.

      90 days to 13 years: 100-300 mg/m^2/day PO bid.

      $\geq$13 years:

          <60 kg: 125 mg q12h (tablets or powder packets) or 167 mg PO q12h (oral susp).

          $\geq$60 kg: 200 mg q12h (tablets or powder packets) or 250 mg PO q12h (oral susp).

      Children >1 year should take drug as two chewable tablets or as powder packets or as suspension to ensure adequate buffering; must be taken on an empty stomach.

      [Powd pkt, buffered: 100, 167, 250 mg; susp: 2, 4 gm bottles (10 mg/mL when mixed with antacid); tabs, chew/buffered: 25, 50, 100, 150, 200 mg].

-Zalcitabine (ddC, Hivid)

      <13 year: 0.005 - 0.01 mg/kg/dose PO q8h.

      $\geq$13 year: 0.75 mg PO q8h.

      [tabs: 0.375, 0.75 mg].

-Stavudine (d4T, Zerit)

      7 mos-15 years: 1-2 mg/kg/day PO bid, max 80 mg/day .

      >15 years or if $\geq$40 kg: 40 mg PO bid.

      [caps: 15, 20, 30, 40 mg; soln: 1 mg/mL].

-Saquinavir (Fortovase, SQV, Invirase)

      1050 mg/m^2/day PO q8h, max 3600 mg/day .

      Diarrhea, abdominal cramps, hyperglycemia. Take with meal to increase absorption.

      [cap: 200 mg].

-Indinavir (IDV, Crixivan)

      350-500 mg/m^2/dose PO q8h.

      Adolescents: 800mg PO q8h.

      Adverse drug reactions include kidney stones, abdominal pain, fatigue. Take on an empty stomach with ample fluids.

      [cap: 200, 400 mg].

-Ritonavir (RTV, Norvir)

      Pediatric: Start at less than 100 mg bid and titrate up over five days to 500-800 mg/m^2/day PO bid.

      Adolescents: start at 300 mg PO bid, increase to full dose of 600 mg PO bid over 5 days.

      Paresthesias, anorexia, increased liver function tests. Take with food.

      [cap: 100 mg; soln: 80 mg/mL].

-Combivir (zidovudine and lamivudine)

      Adolescents: 1 tab PO bid.

[tab: zidovudine 300 mg, lamivudine 150 mg].

Oropharyngeal Candidiasis:

-Ketoconazole (Nizoral) 5-10 mg/kg/day PO qd-bid, max 800 mg/day [tab: 200 mg; suspension may be made] **OR**

-Nystatin susp. Premature infants: 1 mL; infants: 2 mL; children: 5 mL; >12 years: 10 mL. Swish and swallow qid **OR**

-Fluconazole (Diflucan) 6 mg/kg IV or PO loading dose, followed by 3 mg/kg/day PO or IV qd [inj: 2 mg/mL; susp: 10 mg/mL, 40 mg/mL; tabs: 50, 100, 150, 200 mg].

-Itraconazole (Sporanox) 3-5 mg/kg/day PO qd; adolescents may also use oral suspension 10 mL swish/swallow qd-bid [cap: 100 mg; oral soln: 100 mg/10 mL).

Invasive or Disseminated Candidiasis:

-Amphotericin B (Fungizone): test dose of 0.1 mg/kg (max 1 mg), followed by remainder of first days dose if tolerated. Initial dose: 0.25 mg/kg/day; increase by 0.25 mg/kg/day q1-2 days. Usual dose 0.5-1 mg/kg/day; usual max dose 50 mg. Infuse over 2-4 hours.

Pretreatment (except test dose) - Acetaminophen, hydrocortisone, diphenhydramine; give meperidine (Demerol) during infusion if chilling occurs.

-Amphotericin B liposomal (AmBisome) 3-5 mg/kg IV over 2 hrs qd.

-Amphotericin B lipid complex (Abelcet) 5 mg/kg IV over 2 hrs qd.

-Fluconazole (Diflucan) 6-12 mg/kg/day PO/IV qd [inj: 2 mg/mL; susp: 10 mg/mL, 40 mg/mL; tabs: 50, 100, 150, 200 mg]

-Flucytosine (Ancobon) 100-150 mg/kg/day PO q6h [caps: 250, 500 mg; suspension]. Must use in combination with amphotericin B as resistance develops quickly if used alone. Monitor serum levels and adjust dose in renal impairment.

Cryptococcus Neoformans Meningitis:

-Amphotericin B (Fungizone) 1 mg/kg/day IV qd over 2-4h x 8-12 weeks (see test dose and titration, page 59) **OR**

-Fluconazole (Diflucan) 6-12 mg/kg/day IV/PO qd [inj: 2 mg/mL; susp: 10 mg/mL, 40 mg/mL; tabs: 50, 100, 150, 200 mg].

-Flucytosine (Ancobon, 5-FC) 100-150 mg/kg/day PO q6h [caps: 250, 500 mg; suspension].

-Patients infected with HIV who have completed initial therapy for cryptococcosis should receive lifelong maintenance with low-dose fluconazole.

Herpes Simplex Infections in Immunocompromised Host:

-Acyclovir (Zovirax) 15-30 mg/kg/day or 250-500 mg/m^2/dose IV q8h for 7-14 days (infuse each dose over 1 hr) or 500 mg/m^2/dose PO 4-5 times daily.

Herpes Simplex Encephalitis:

-Acyclovir (Zovirax) 30 mg/kg/day or 500 mg/m^2/dose IV q8h (infuse each dose over 1 hr).

Herpes Varicella Zoster:
  -Acyclovir (Zovirax) 30 mg/kg/day or 500 mg/m^2/dose IV q8h for 10 days (infuse each dose over 1 hr).

Cytomegalovirus Infections:
  -Ganciclovir (Cytovene) children >3 months-adults: 10 mg/kg/day IV over 1-2h q12h x 14-21 days, then maintenance 5 mg/kg/day IV qd for 5-7 days per week.

Toxoplasmosis:
  -Pyrimethamine (Daraprim) 2 mg/kg/day PO qd x 3 days, then 1 mg/kg/day PO q24h, max 25 mg/day [tab: 25 mg] and folinic acid 5-10 mg PO q3 days [tabs: 5, 15, 25 mg] **AND**
  -Sulfadiazine 100-200 mg/kg/day PO qid x 3-4 weeks, max 6 gm/day [tab: 500 mg; suspension]. Take with ample fluids.

Disseminated Histoplasmosis or Coccidiomycosis:
  -Amphotericin B (Fungizone) 1 mg/kg/day IV qd over 2-4h for ≥6 weeks (see test dose and titration, page 59).

Mycobacterium Avium Complex (MAC):
  -Azithromycin (Zithromax) 10-20 mg/kg/day PO qd, max 500 mg [cap: 250 mg; susp: 100 mg/5 mL, 200 mg/5 mL; tabs: 250, 600 mg] **AND**
  -Rifabutin (Mycobutin)
    6-12 year: 5 mg/kg/day PO qd, max 300 mg/day
    >12 year: 300 mg/day PO qd
    [cap: 150 mg] **OR**
  -Ethambutol (Myambutol) 15-25 mg/kg/day PO qd, max 1 gm /day [tab: 100, 400 mg] **OR**
  -Rifampin (Rifadin) 10-20 mg/kg/day PO q12-24h, max 600 mg/day [caps: 150, 300 mg; suspension].
  Single drug therapy results in frequent development of MAC antimicrobial resistance. Patients with HIV should continue treatment at full therapeutic doses for life.

Septic Arthritis

1. **Admit to:**
2. **Diagnosis:** Septic arthritis.
3. **Condition:**
4. **Vital signs:** Call MD if:
5. **Activity:** No weight bearing on infected joint.
6. **Nursing:** Warm compresses prn. Consent for arthrocentesis.
7. **Diet:**
8. **IV Fluids:**

9. Special Medications:

Empiric Therapy for Infants 1-6 months (strep, staph, gram neg, gono-coccus):

-Nafcillin (Nafcil) or oxacillin (Bactocill, Prostaphlin) 100 mg/kg/day IV/IM q6h **AND**

-Cefotaxime (Claforan) 100 mg/kg/day IV/IM q6h **OR**

-Gentamicin (Garamycin) or tobramycin (Nebcin) (normal renal function): 7.5 mg/kg/day IV/IM q8h.

Empiric Therapy for Patients Age 6 months-4 year (H influenzae, strepto-cocci, staphylococcus):

-Cefuroxime (Zinacef) 100-150 mg/kg/day IV/IM q8h (preferred for H flu coverage until culture results available) **AND/OR**

-Nafcillin (Nafcil) or oxacillin (Bactocill) 100-200 mg/kg/day IV/IM q6h.

Empiric Therapy for Children Older than 4 Years (staph, strep):

-Nafcillin (Nafcil) or oxacillin (Bactocill, Prostaphlin) 150 mg/kg/day IV/IM q6h, max 12 gm/day **OR**

-Vancomycin (Vancocin) (MRSA) 40-60 mg/kg/day IV q6-8h, max 4 gm/day.

10. Symptomatic Medications:

-Acetaminophen and codeine 0.5-1 mg codeine/kg/dose PO q4-6h prn pain [elixir per 5 mL: codeine 12 mg, acetaminophen 120 mg].

-Ibuprofen (Children's Advil) 5-10 mg/kg/dose PO q6-8 hrs prn fever.

11. Extras and X-rays: X-ray views of joint, CXR. Orthopedics and infectious disease consults. CT scan.

12. Labs: CBC, blood culture and sensitivity x 2, PPD, ESR, UA. Antibiotic levels.

Synovial fluid:

Tube 1 - Gram stain, culture and sensitivity.

Tube 2 - Glucose, protein, pH.

Tube 3 - Cell count.

Appendicitis

1. Admit to:

2. Diagnosis: Appendicitis.

3. Condition: Guarded.

4. Vital signs: Call MD if:

5. Activity:

6. Nursing: Inputs and outputs, daily weights; cooling measures prn temp >38°C. Age appropriate pain scale.

7. Diet:

8. IV Fluids: Isotonic fluids at maintenance rate.

9. Special Medications:

-Ampicillin 100 mg/kg/day IV/IM q6h, max 12 gm/day **AND**

-Gentamicin (Garamycin):

    30 days-5 year: 7.5 mg/kg/day IV/IM q8h.

    5-10 year: 6.0 mg/kg/day IV/IM q8h.

    >10 year: 5.0 mg/kg/day IV/IM q8h **AND**

-Metronidazole (Flagyl) 30 mg/kg/day q6h, max 4 gm/day

OR (non-perforated)

-Cefotetan (Cefotan) 40-80 mg/kg/day IM/IV q12h, max 6 gm/day **OR**

-Cefoxitin (Mefoxin) 100 mg/kg/day IM/IV q6-8h, max 12 gm/day

10. Symptomatic Medications:

-Ibuprofen 5-10 mg/kg/dose PO q6-8h prn **OR**

-Acetaminophen 15 mg/kg PO/PR q4h prn temp >38°C or pain.

11. Extras and X-rays: Abdominal ultrasound, abdominal x-ray series.

12. Labs: CBC, SMA 7, blood culture and sensitivity, antibiotic levels.

Lower Urinary Tract Infection

1. Admit to:

2. Diagnosis: UTI

3. Condition:

4. Vital signs: Call MD if:

5. Activity:

6. Nursing: Inputs and outputs

7. Diet:

8. IV Fluids:

9. Special Medications:

Lower Urinary Tract Infection:

-Cefpodoxime (Vantin) 10 mg/kg/day PO q12h, max 800 mg/day [susp: 50 mg/5 mL, 100 mg/5 mL; tabs: 100, 200 mg] **OR**

-Cefprozil (Cefzil) 30 mg/kg/day PO q12h, max 1 gm/day [susp: 125 mg/5 mL, 250 mg/5 mL; tabs: 250, 500 mg] **OR**

-Cefixime (Suprax) 8 mg/kg/d PO qd-bid [susp: 100 mg/5 mL, tab: 200,400 mg] **OR**

-Cefuroxime (Ceftin) 125-500 mg PO q12h [125, 250, 500 mg] **OR**

-Amoxicillin/clavulanate (Augmentin) 40 mg of amoxicillin kg/day PO q8h [susp: amoxicillin 125 mg/clavulanate/5 mL; tab: amoxicillin 250 mg/clavulanate; amoxicillin 500 mg/clavulanate] **OR**

-Trimethoprim/sulfamethoxazole (Bactrim, Septra) 6-10 mg/kg/day TMP PO q12h, max 320 mg TMP/day [susp per 5 mL: TMP 40 mg, SMX 200 mg; tab, SS: 80 mg/400 mg; tab, DS: 160 mg/800 mg].

Prophylactic Therapy:

-Trimethoprim/sulfamethoxazole (Bactrim, Septra) 2 mg TMP/kg/day and 10 mg SMX/kg/day PO qhs [susp per 5 mL: TMP 40 mg/SMX 200 mg; tab DS: TMP 160 mg/SMX 800 mg; tab SS: TMP 80mg/SMX 400 mg] **OR**

-Sulfisoxazole (Gantrisin) 10-20 mg/kg/day PO q12h [500 mg/5 mL; tab: 500 mg].

10. **Symptomatic Medications:**

-Phenazopyridine (Pyridium), children 6-12 years: 12 mg/kg/day PO tid (max 200 mg/dose); >12 years: 100-200 mg PO tid x 2 days prn dysuria [tabs: 100, 200 mg].

11. **Extras and X-rays:** Renal ultrasound. Voiding cystourethrogram 3 weeks after infection. Radiological work up on all children <1 year of age.

12. **Labs:** CBC, SMA 7. UA with micro, urine Gram stain, culture and sensitivity. Blood culture and sensitivity.

Pyelonephritis

1. **Admit to:**
2. **Diagnosis:** Pyelonephritis.
3. **Condition:**
4. **Vital signs:** Call MD if:
5. **Activity:**
6. **Nursing:** Inputs and outputs, daily weights.
7. **Diet:**
8. **IV Fluids:**
9. **Special Medications:**

-If <1 week old, see suspected sepsis, pages 41, 117.

-Ampicillin 100 mg/kg/day IV/IM q6h, max 12 gm/day **AND**

-Gentamicin (Garamycin) or Tobramycin (Nebcin):

    30 days-5 year: 7.5 mg/kg/day IV/IM q8h.

    5-10 year: 6.0 mg/kg/day IV/IM q8h.

    >10 year: 5.0 mg/kg/day IV/IM q8h **OR**

-Cefotaxime (Claforan) 100 mg/kg/day IV/IM q8h, max 12 gm/day.

10. **Symptomatic Medications:**

-Acetaminophen (Tylenol) 10-15 mg/kg PO/PR q4-6h prn temp >38°.

11. **Extras and X-rays:** Renal ultrasound.

12. **Labs:** CBC, SMA-7. UA with micro, urine culture and sensitivity. Blood culture and sensitivity x 2.

Osteomyelitis

1. **Admit to:**
2. **Diagnosis:** Osteomyelitis.
3. **Condition:**
4. **Vital signs:** Call MD if:
5. **Activity:**
6. **Nursing:** Keep involved extremity elevated. Consent for osteotomy.
7. **Diet:**
8. **IV Fluids:**
9. **Special Medications:**

Children ≤3 years (H flu, strep, staph):
   -Cefuroxime (Zinacef) 100-150 mg/kg/day IV/IM q8h, max 9 gm/day.

Children >3 years (staph, strep, H flu):
   -Nafcillin (Nafcil) or oxacillin (Bactophill) 100-150 mg/kg/day IV/IM q6h, max 12 gm/day **OR**
   -Cefotaxime (Claforan) 100-150 mg/kg/day IV/IM q8h, max 12 gm/day **OR**
   -Cefazolin (Ancef) 100 mg/kg/day IV/IM q6-8h, max 6 gm/day **OR**
   -Cefuroxime (Zinacef) 100-150 mg/kg/day IV/IM q8h, max 9 gm/day.

Postoperative or Traumatic (staph, gram neg, Pseudomonas):
   -Ticarcillin/Clavulanate (Timentin) 200-300 mg/kg/day of ticarcillin IV/IM q6-8h, max 24 gm/day **OR**
   -Vancomycin (Vancocin) 40-60 mg/kg/day IV q6-8h, max 4 gm/day **AND**
   -Ceftazidime (Fortaz) 150 mg/kg/day IV/IM q8h, max 12 gm/day **OR**
   -Nafcillin (Nafcil) or oxacillin (Bactocill) 150 mg/kg/day IV/IM q6h, max 12 gm/day **AND**
   -Tobramycin (Nebcin)
      30 days-5 year: 7.5 mg/kg/day IV/IM q8h.
      5-10 year: 6.0 mg/kg/day IV/IM q8h.
      >10 year: 5.0 mg/kg/day IV q8h.

Chronic Osteomyelitis (staphylococcal):
   -Dicloxacillin (Dycill, Dynapen, Pathocil) 75-100 mg/kg/day PO q6h, max 2 gm/day [caps: 125, 250, 500 mg; susp: 62.5 mg/5 mL] **OR**
   -Cephalexin (Keflex) 50-100 mg/kg/day PO q6-12h, max 4 gm/day [caps: 250, 500 mg; drops 100 mg/mL; susp 125 mg/5 mL, 250 mg/5 mL; tabs: 500 mg, 1 gm].

10. **Symptomatic Medications:**
   -Acetaminophen (Tylenol) 10-15 mg/kg PO/PR q4-6h prn temp >38°.
11. **Extras and X-rays:** Bone scan, multiple X-ray views, CT. Orthopedic and infectious disease consultations.
12. **Labs:** CBC, SMA 7, blood culture and sensitivity x 3, ESR, sickle prep, UA, culture and sensitivity, antibiotic levels, serum bacteriocidal titers.

Otitis Media

Acute Otitis Media (S pneumoniae, non-typable H flu, M catarrhalis, Staph a, group A strep):

-Amoxicillin (Amoxil) 80 to 90 mg/kg per day divided bid
[caps: 250, 500 mg; drops: 50 mg/mL; susp; 125 mg/5mL, 200 mg/5mL, 250 mg/5mL, 400 mg/5mL; tabs: 500, 875 mg; tabs, chew: 125, 200, 250, 400 mg] **OR**

-Cefdinir (Omnicef) (14 mg/kg per day in 1 or 2 doses) [cap: 300 mg, susp: 125 mg/5 mL] **OR**

-Cefpodoxime (Vantin) 10 mg/kg/day PO bid, max 800 mg/day
[susp: 50 mg/5 mL, 100 mg/5 mL; tabs: 100, 200 mg] **OR**

-Cefuroxime axetil (Ceftin) tab: child: 125-250 mg PO bid; adult: 250-500 mg PO bid; susp: 30 mg/kg/day PO q12h, max 500 mg/day
[susp: 125 mg/5 mL; tabs 125, 250, 500 mg] **OR**

-Erythromycin/sulfisoxazole (Pediazole) 1 mL/kg/day PO qid or 50-150 mg/kg per day of erythromycin PO qid, max 50 mL/day
[susp per 5 mL: erythromycin 200 mg/sulfisoxazole 600 mg] **OR**

-Azithromycin (Zithromax)
Children ≥2 years: 10 mg/kg/day PO qd x 5 days, max 500 mg/day
≥16 years: 500 mg PO on day 1, 250 mg PO qd on days 2-5
[cap: 250 mg; susp: 100 mg/5mL, 200 mg/5mL; tabs: 250, 600 mg]
OR

-Clarithromycin (Biaxin) 15 mg/kg/day PO bid, max 1 gm/day
[susp: 125 mg/5 mL, 250 mg/5 mL; tabs: 250, 500 mg] **OR**

-Amoxicillin/clavulanate (Augmentin BID) 90 mg/kg/day of amoxicillin PO bid x 7-10d, max 500 mg/dose [susp: 200 mg/5mL, 400 mg/5mL; tab: 875 mg; tab, chew: 200, 400 mg] **OR**

-Cefixime (Suprax) 8 mg/kg/day PO bid-qd, max 400 mg/day
[susp: 100 mg/5 mL; tabs: 200, 400 mg] **OR**

-Loracarbef (Lorabid) 30 mg/kg/day PO bid, max 400 mg/day
[caps: 200, 400 mg; susp: 100 mg/5 mL, 200 mg/5mL] **OR**

-Cefprozil (Cefzil) 30 mg/kg/day PO bid, max 1gm/day
[susp: 125 mg/5 mL, 250 mg/5 mL; tabs: 250 mg, 500 mg] **OR**

-Ceftriaxone (Rocephin) 50 mg/kg IM x one dose, max 2000 mg

-Trimethoprim/sulfamethoxazole (Bactrim, Septra) 6-8 mg/kg/day of TMP PO bid, max 320 mg TMP/day
[susp per 5 mL: TMP 40 mg/SMX 200 mg; tab DS: TMP 160 mg/SMX 800 mg; tab SS: TMP 80mg/SMX 400 mg].

Prophylactic Therapy (≥3 episodes in 6 months):
Therapy reserved for control of recurrent acute otitis media, defined as three or more episodes per 6 months or 4 or more episodes per 12 months.

-Sulfisoxazole (Gantrisin) 50 mg/kg/day PO qhs
[tab 500 mg; susp 500 mg/5 mL] **OR**

-Amoxicillin (Amoxil) 20 mg/kg/day PO qhs
   [caps: 250,500 mg; drops: 50 mg/mL; susp; 125 mg/5mL, 200 mg/5mL, 250 mg/5mL, 400 mg/5mL; tabs: 500, 875 mg; tabs, chew: 125, 200, 250, 400mg] **OR**
-Trimethoprim/sulfamethoxazole (Bactrim, Septra) 4 mg/kg/day of TMP PO qhs
   [susp per 5 mL: TMP 40 mg/SMX 200 mg; tab DS: TMP 160 mg/SMX 800 mg; tab SS: TMP 80mg/SMX 400 mg]

Symptomatic Therapy:

-Ibuprofen (Advil) 5-10 mg/kg/dose PO q6-8 hrs prn fever
   [suspension: 100 mg/5 mL, tabs: 200, 300, 400, 600, 800 mg] **AND/OR**
-Acetaminophen (Tylenol) 10-15 mg/kg/dose PO/PR q4-6h prn fever
   [tabs: 325, 500 mg; chewable tabs: 80 mg; caplets: 160 mg, 500 mg; drops: 80 mg/0.8 mL; elixir: 120 mg/5 mL, 130 mg/5 mL, 160 mg/5 mL, 325 mg/5 mL; caplet, ER: 650 mg; suppositories: 120, 325, 650 mg].
-Benzocaine/antipyrine (Auralgan otic): fill ear canal with 2-4 drops; moisten cotton pledget and place in external ear; repeat every 1-2 hours prn pain
   [soln, otic: Antipyrine 5.4%, benzocaine 1.4% in 10 mL and 15 mL bottles]

Extras and X rays: Aspiration tympanocentesis, tympanogram; audiometry.

Otitis Externa

Otitis Externa (Pseudomonas, gram negatives, proteus):

-Polymyxin B/neomycin/hydrocortisone (Cortisporin otic susp or solution) 2-4 drops in ear canal tid-qid x 5-7 days.
   [otic soln or susp per mL: neomycin sulfate 5 mg; polymyxin B sulfate 10,000 units; hydrocortisone 10 mg in 10 mL bottles)].
   The suspension is preferred. The solution should not be used if the ear-drum is perforated.

Malignant Otitis Externa in Diabetes (Pseudomonas):

-Ceftazidime (Fortaz) 100-150 mg/kg/day IV/IM q8h, max 12gm/day **OR**
-Piperacillin (Pipracil) or ticarcillin (Ticar) 200-300 mg/kg/day IV/IM q4-6h, max 24gm/day **OR**
-Tobramycin (Nebcin)
   30 days-5 year: 7.5 mg/kg/day IV/IM q8h.
   5-10 year: 6.0 mg/kg/day IV/IM q8h.
   >10 year: 5.0 mg/kg/day IV q8h.

Tonsillopharyngitis

Streptococcal Pharyngitis:
-Penicillin V (Pen Vee K) 25-50 mg/kg/day PO qid x 10 days, max 3 gm/day
[susp: 125 mg/5 mL, 250 mg/5 mL; tabs: 125, 250, 500 mg] **OR**
-Amoxicillin (Amoxil) 40 mg/kg/day PO tid, max 3 gm/day [caps: 250,500 mg;
drops: 50 mg/mL; susp; 125 mg/5mL, 200 mg/5mL, 250 mg/5mL, 400
mg/5mL; tabs: 500, 875 mg; tabs, chew: 125, 200, 250 , 400mg]
-Penicillin G benzathine (Bicillin LA) 25,000-50,000 U/kg (max 1.2 MU) IM x
1 dose **OR**
-Azithromycin (Zithromax) 10 mg/kg/day PO qd x 5 days, max 500 mg/day
[cap: 250 mg; susp: 100 mg/5mL, 200 mg/5mL; tabs: 250, 600 mg] **OR**
-Clarithromycin (Biaxin)15 mg/kg/day PO bid, max 1 gm/day
[susp 125 mg/5 mL, 250 mg/5 mL; tabs: 250, 500 mg] **OR**
-Erythromycin (penicillin-allergic patients) 40 mg/kg/day PO qid x 10 days,
max 2 gm/day
Erythromycin ethylsuccinate (EryPed, EES)
[susp: 200 mg/5 mL, 400 mg/5 mL; tab: 400 mg; tab, chew: 200 mg]
Erythromycin base (E-Mycin, Ery-Tab, Eryc)
[cap, DR: 250 mg; tabs: 250, 333, 500 mg]

Refractory Pharyngitis:
-Amoxicillin/clavulanate (Augmentin)
40 mg/kg/day of amoxicillin PO q8h x 7-10d, max 500 mg/dose
[susp: 125 mg/5 mL, 250 mg/5 mL; tabs: 250, 500 mg; tabs, chew: 125,
250 mg] **OR**
-Dicloxacillin (Dycill, Dynapen, Pathocil)
50 mg/kg/day PO qid, max 2 gm/day
[caps 125, 250, 500; elixir 62.5 mg/5 mL] **OR**
-Cephalexin (Keflex)
50 mg/kg/day PO qid-tid, max 4 gm/day
[caps: 250, 500 mg; drops 100 mg/mL; susp 125 mg/5 mL, 250 mg/5 mL;
tabs: 500 mg, 1 gm].

Prophylaxis (5 strep infections in 6 months):
-Penicillin V Potassium (Pen Vee K)
40 mg/kg/day PO bid, max 3 gm/day
[susp 125 mg/5 mL, 250 mg/5 mL; tabs: 125, 250, 500 mg].

Retropharyngeal Abscess (strep, anaerobes, E corrodens):
-Clindamycin (Cleocin) 25-40 mg/kg/day IV/IM q6-8h, max 4.8 gm/day **OR**
-Nafcillin (Nafcil) or oxacillin (Bactocill, Prostaphlin) 100-150 mg/kg/day IV/IM
q6h, max 12 gm/day **AND**
-Cefuroxime (Zinacef) 75-100 mg/kg/day IV/IM q8h, max 9 gm/day

Labs: Throat culture, rapid antigen test; PA lateral and neck films; CXR.
Otolaryngology consult for incision and drainage.

Epiglottitis

1. **Admit to:** Pediatric intensive care unit.
2. **Diagnosis:** Epiglottitis
3. **Condition:**
4. **Vital Signs:** Call MD if:
5. **Activity:**
6. **Nursing:** Pulse oximeter. Keep head of bed elevated, allow patient to sit; curved blade laryngoscope, tracheostomy tray and oropharyngeal tube at bedside. Respiratory isolation.
7. **Diet:** NPO
8. **IV Fluids:**
9. **Special Medications:**
   -Oxygen, humidified, blow-by; keep sat >92%.
Antibiotics:
   -Ceftriaxone (Rocephin) 50 mg/kg/day IV/IM qd, max 2 gm/day **OR**
   -Cefuroxime (Zinacef) 100-150 mg/kg/day IV/IM q8h, max 9 gm/day **OR**
   -Cefotaxime (Claforan) 100-150 mg/kg/day IV/IM q6-8h, max 12 gm/day
10. **Extras and X-rays:** CXR PA and LAT, lateral neck. Otolaryngology consult.
11. **Labs:** CBC, CBG/ABG. Blood culture and sensitivity, latex agglutination; UA, urine antigen screen.

Sinusitis

Treatment of Sinusitis (S. pneumoniae, H flu, M catarrhalis, group A strep, anaerobes):
   -Treat for 14-21 days.
   -Amoxicillin (Amoxil) 80 to 90 mg/kg per day divided bid [caps: 250,500 mg; drops: 50 mg/mL; susp; 125 mg/5mL, 200 mg/5mL, 250 mg/5mL, 400 mg/5mL; tabs: 500, 875 mg; tabs, chew: 125, 200, 250 , 400mg] **OR**
   -Azithromycin (Zithromax)
      Children ≥2 years: 12 mg/kg/day PO qd x 5 days, max 500 mg/day
      ≥16 years: 500 mg PO on day 1, 250 mg PO qd on days 2-5
      [cap: 250 mg; susp: 100 mg/5mL, 200 mg/5mL; tab: 250, 600 mg] **OR**
   -Trimethoprim/sulfamethoxazole (Bactrim, Septra) 6-8 mg/kg/day of TMP PO bid, max 320 mg TMP/day
      [susp per 5 mL: TMP 40 mg/SMX 200 mg; tab DS: TMP 160 mg/SMX 800 mg; tab SS: TMP 80mg/SMX 400 mg] **OR**
   -Erythromycin/sulfisoxazole (Pediazole) 1 mL/kg/day PO qid or 40-50 mg/kg/day of erythromycin PO qid, max 2 gm erythromycin/day

[susp per 5 mL: Erythromycin 200 mg, sulfisoxazole 600 mg] **OR**
-Amoxicillin/clavulanate (Augmentin) 40 mg/kg/day of amoxicillin PO tid, max 500 mg/dose

[elixir 125 mg/5 mL, 250 mg/5 mL; tabs: 250, 500 mg; tabs, chew: 125, 250 mg] **OR**
-Amoxicillin/clavulanate (Augmentin BID)

40 mg/kg/day PO bid, max 875 mg (amoxicillin)/dose

[susp: 200 mg/5 mL, 400 mg/5 mL; tab: 875 mg; tabs, chew: 200, 400 mg] **OR**
-Cefuroxime axetil (Ceftin)

tab: child: 125-250 mg PO bid; adult: 250-500 mg PO bid

susp: 30 mg/kg/day PO qid, max 500 mg/day

[susp: 125 mg/5 mL; tabs: 125, 250, 500 mg]

Helicobacter Pylori

1. **Admit to:**
2. **Diagnosis:** Helicobacter pylori.
3. **Condition:** Guarded.
4. **Vital signs:** Call MD if:
5. **Activity:**
6. **Nursing:**
7. **Diet:**
8. **IV Fluids:** Isotonic fluids at maintenance rate.
9. **Special Medications:**
   Triple-drug regimens are more effective for eradication than two-drug regimens.

Antimicrobial Agents

-Amoxicillin (Amoxil) 25-50 mg/kg/day PO bid-tid (max 3 gm/day)

[caps: 250,500 mg; drops: 50 mg/mL; susp; 125 mg/5mL, 200 mg/5mL, 250 mg/5mL, 400 mg/5mL; tabs: 500, 875 mg; tabs, chew: 125, 200, 250mg , 400mg]
-Tetracycline (Achromycin) **>8 years only**

25-50 mg/kg/day PO q6h, max 2 gm/day

[caps: 100, 250, 500 mg; susp: 125 mg/5 mL; tabs: 250, 500 mg]
-Metronidazole (Flagyl): 35-50 mg/kg/day PO q8h, max 2250 mg/day [tabs: 250, 500 mg; suspension]
-Clarithromycin (Biaxin)15 mg/kg/day PO bid, max 1 gm/day

[susp 125 mg/5 mL, 250 mg/5 mL; tabs: 250, 500 mg]

H-2 Blockers

-Ranitidine (Zantac) 4-6 mg/kg/day PO q12h [liquid: 15 mg/mL; tabs: 75, 150, 300 mg]

Proton Pump Inhibitors
  -Lansoprazole (Prevacid)
     <0 kg: 7.5 mg PO qd
     10-20 kg: 15 mg PO qd
     > 20 kg: 30 mg PO qd
     Adolescents: 15-30 mg PO qd
     [caps: 15, 30 mg; suspension can be made by dissolving the capsules in sodium bicarbonate. The capsule may also be opened and mixed with applesauce].
  -Omeprazole (Prilosec)
     0.3-3 mg/kg/day PO qd (max 20 mg/day)
     [caps: 10, 20, 40 mg; suspension is made by dissolving the capsule in sodium bicarbonate]
Bismuth subsalicylate (Pepto-Bismol)
  ≤10 years: 262 mg PO qid
  >10 years: 524 mg PO qid
  [cap: 262 mg; liquid: 262 mg/15 mL, 525 mg/15 mL; tab, chew: 262 mg].
10. **Symptomatic Medications:**
   -Acetaminophen 15 mg/kg PO/PR q4h prn temp >38°C or pain.
11. **Extras and X-rays:** Endoscopy, gastric biopsy.
12. **Labs:** Gastric biopsy, ELISA IgG for H. pylori, stool ELISA for H. pylori antigen, urea breath test.

Active Pulmonary Tuberculosis

1. **Admit to:**
2. **Diagnosis:** Active Pulmonary Tuberculosis
3. **Condition:**
4. **Vital signs:**
5. **Activity:**
6. **Nursing:** Respiratory isolation.
7. **Diet:**
8. **Special Medications:**
Pulmonary Infection:

Six-Month Regimen: Two months of isoniazid, rifampin and pyrazinamide daily, followed by four months of isoniazid and rifampin daily **OR**
   Two months of isoniazid, rifampin and pyrazinamide daily, followed by four months of isoniazid and rifampin twice weekly.

Nine-Month Regimen (for hilar adenopathy only): Nine months of isoniazid and rifampin daily **OR** one month of isoniazid and rifampin daily, followed by 8 months of isoniazid and rifampin twice weekly.

Anti-tuberculosis Agents			
Drug	Daily Dose	Twice Weekly Dose	Dosage Forms
Isoniazid (Laniazid)	10-15 mg/kg/day PO qd, max 300 mg	20-30 mg/kg PO, max 900 mg	Tab: 50, 100, 300 mg Syrup: 10 mg/mL
Rifampin (Rifadin)	10-20 mg/kg/day PO qd, max 600 mg	10-20 mg/kg, max 600 mg	Cap: 150, 300 mg suspension
Pyrazinamide	20-40 mg/kg PO qd, max 2000 mg	50 mg/kg PO, max 2000 mg	Tab: 500 mg suspension
Ethambutol (Myambutol)	15-25 mg/kg/day PO qd, max 2500 mg	50 mg/kg PO, max 2500 mg	Tab: 100, 400 mg
Streptomycin	20-40 mg/kg IM qd, max 1 gm	20-40 mg/kg IM, max 1 gm	Inj: 400 mg/mL, IM only

-Directly observed therapy should be considered for all patients. All household contacts should be tested.

Tuberculosis Prophylaxis for Skin Test Conversion:
  -Isoniazid-susceptible: Isoniazid (Laniazid) 10 mg/kg/day (max 300 mg) PO qd x 6-9 months.
  -Isoniazid-resistant: Rifampin (Rifadin) 10 mg/kg/day (max 600 mg) PO qd for 9 months.

9. **Extras and X-rays:** CXR PA, LAT.
10. **Labs:** CBC, SMA7, liver panel, HIV antibody, ABG. First AM sputum for AFB x 3 (drug-sensitivity tests on first isolate). Gastric aspirates for AFB qAM x 3. UA, urine AFB.

Cellulitis

1. **Admit to:**
2. **Diagnosis:** Cellulitis.
3. **Condition:**
4. **Vital signs:** Call MD if
5. **Activity:**
6. **Nursing:** Keep affected extremity elevated; warm compresses tid prn. Monitor area of infection.
7. **Diet:**
8. **IV Fluids:**
9. **Special Medications:**

Empiric Therapy for Extremity Cellulitis:

-Nafcillin (Nafcil) or oxacillin (Bactocill, Prostaphlin) 100-200 mg/kg/day/IV/IM q4-6h, max 12 gm/day **OR**

-Cefazolin (Ancef) 75-100 mg/kg/day IV/IM q6-8h, max 6 gm/day **OR**

-Cefoxitin (Mefoxin) 100-160 mg/kg/day IV/IM q6h, max 12 gm/day **OR**

-Ticarcillin/clavulanate (Timentin) 200-300 mg/kg/day IV/IM q6-8h, max 24 gm/day **OR**

-Dicloxacillin (Dycill, Dynapen, Pathocil) 50-100 mg/kg/day PO qid, max 2 gm/day [caps: 125, 250, 500 mg; susp: 62.5 mg/5 mL].

Cheek/Buccal Cellulitis (H flu):

-Cefuroxime (Zinacef) 100-150 mg/kg/day IV/IM q8h, max 9 gm/day **OR**

-Cefotaxime (Claforan) 100-150 mg/kg/day IV/IM q6-8h, max 12 gm/day

Periorbital Cellulitis (H. flu, pneumococcus):

-Cefuroxime (Zinacef) 100-150 mg/kg/day IV/IM q8h, max 9 gm/day **OR**

-Cefuroxime axetil (Ceftin)

    tab: child: 125-250 mg PO bid; adult: 250-500 mg PO bid

    susp: 30 mg/kg/day PO qid, max 500 mg/day

    [susp: 125 mg/5 mL; tabs: 125, 250, 500 mg]

10. **Symptomatic Medications:**

-Acetaminophen and codeine, 0.5-1 mg codeine/kg/dose PO q4-6h prn pain [elixir per 5 mL: codeine 12 mg, acetaminophen 120 mg].

11. **Extras and X-rays:** X-ray views of site.

12. **Labs:** CBC, SMA 7, blood culture and sensitivity. Leading edge aspirate, Gram stain, culture and sensitivity; UA, urine culture.

Impetigo, Scalded Skin Syndrome, and Staphylococcal Scarlet Fever

1. **Admit to:**
2. **Diagnosis:** Impetigo, scalded skin syndrome or staphylococcal scarlet fever.
3. **Condition:**
4. **Vital signs:** Call MD if:
5. **Activity:**
6. **Nursing:** Warm compresses tid prn.
7. **Diet:**
8. **IV Fluids:**
9. **Special Medications:**

-Nafcillin (Nafcil) or oxacillin (Bactocill, Prostaphlin) 100-200 mg/kg/day IV/IM q4-6h, max 12 gm/day **OR**

-Dicloxacillin (Dycill, Dynapen, Pathocil) 25-50 mg/kg/day PO qid x 5-7days, max 2 gm/day [caps 125, 250, 500 mg; elixir 62.5 mg/5 mL] **OR**

-Cephalexin (Keflex) 25-50 mg/kg/day PO qid, max 4 gm/day [caps: 250, 500 mg; drops 100 mg/mL; susp 125 mg/5 mL, 250 mg/5 mL; tabs: 500 mg, 1 gm] **OR**

-Loracarbef (Lorabid) 30 mg/kg/day PO bid, max 800 mg/day [caps: 200, 400 mg; susp: 100 mg/5 mL, 200 mg/5mL] **OR**

-Cefpodoxime (Vantin) 10 mg/kg/day PO bid, max 800 mg/day [susp: 50 mg/5 mL, 100 mg/5 mL; tabs: 100 mg, 200 mg] **OR**

-Cefprozil (Cefzil) 30 mg/kg/day PO bid, max 1 gm/day [susp 125 mg/5 mL, 250 mg/5 mL; tabs: 250, 500 mg] **OR**

-Vancomycin (Vancocin) 40 mg/kg/day IV q6-8h, max 4 gm/day.

10. **Symptomatic Medications:**
-Acetaminophen and codeine, 0.5-1 mg codeine/kg/dose PO q4-6h prn pain [elixir per 5 mL: codeine 12 mg, acetaminophen 120 mg].

11. **Labs:** CBC, SMA 7, blood culture and sensitivity. Drainage fluid for Gram stain, culture and sensitivity; UA.

Tetanus

History of One or Two Primary Immunizations or Unknown:
Low-risk wound - Tetanus toxoid 0.5 mL IM.

Tetanus prone - Tetanus toxoid 0.5 mL IM, plus tetanus immunoglobulin (TIG) 250 U IM.

Three Primary Immunizations and 10 years or more Since Last Booster:
Low-risk wound - Tetanus toxoid, 0.5 mL IM.

Tetanus prone - Tetanus toxoid, 0.5 mL IM.

Three Primary Immunizations and 5-10 years Since Last Booster:
Low-risk wound - None

Tetanus prone - Tetanus toxoid 0.5 mL IM.

Three Primary Immunizations and ≤5 years Since Last Booster:
Low-risk wound - None

Tetanus prone - None

Treatment of Clostridium Tetani Infection:
-Tetanus immune globulin (TIG): single dose of 3,000 to 6,000 U IM (consider immune globulin intravenous if TIG is not available). Part of the TIG dose may be infiltrated locally around the wound. Keep wound clean and débrided.

-Penicillin G 100,000 U/kg/day IV q4-6h, max 24 MU/day x 10-14 days **OR**

-Metronidazole (Flagyl) 30 mg/kg/day PO/IV q6h, max 4 gm/day x 10-14 days

Pelvic Inflammatory Disease

1. **Admit to:**
2. **Diagnosis:** Pelvic Inflammatory Disease (PID).
3. **Condition:**
4. **Vital signs:** Call MD if:
5. **Activity:**
6. **Nursing:**
7. **Diet:**
8. **IV Fluids:**
9. **Special Medications:**

Adolescent Outpatients

- Ofloxacin (Floxin, 400 mg PO twice daily) or levofloxacin (Levaquin, 500 mg once daily) with or without metronidazole (Flagyl, 500 mg twice daily) for 14 days. **OR**
- Ceftriaxone (Rocephin, 250 mg IM), cefoxitin (Mefoxin, 2 g IM plus probenecid 1 g orally), or another parenteral third-generation cephalosporin, followed by doxycycline (100 mg orally twice daily) with or without metronidazole for 14 days. Quinolones are not recommended to treat gonorrhea acquired in California or Hawaii. If the patient may have acquired the disease in Asia, Hawaii, or California, cefixime or ceftriaxone should be used **OR**
- Azithromycin (Zithromax, 1 g PO for Chlamydia coverage) and amoxicillin/clavulanate (Amoxicillin, 875 mg PO) once by directly observed therapy, followed by amoxicillin/clavulanate (Amoxicillin, 875 mg PO BID) for 7 to 10 days.

Adolescent Inpatients

- Cefotetan (Cefotan), 2 g IV Q12h, or cefoxitin (Mefoxin, 2 g IV Q6h) plus doxycycline (100 mg IV or PO Q12h) **OR**
- Clindamycin (Cleocin), 900 mg IV Q8h, plus gentamicin (1-1.5 mg/kg IV q8h)
- Ampicillin-sulbactam (Unasyn), 3 g IV Q6h plus doxycycline (100 mg IV or PO Q12h)
- Parenteral administration of antibiotics should be continued for 24 hours after clinical response, followed by doxycycline (100 mg PO BID) or clindamycin (Cleocin, 450 mg PO QID) for a total of 14 days.
- Levofloxacin (Levaquin), 500 mg IV Q24h, plus metronidazole (Flagyl, 500 mg IV Q8h). With this regimen, azithromycin (Zithromax, 1 g PO once) should be given as soon as the patient is tolerating oral intake.

Gonorrhea in Children less than 45 kg:

Uncomplicated Vulvovaginitis, Cervicitis, Urethritis, Proctitis, or Pharyngitis:

- Ceftriaxone (Rocephin) 125 mg IM x 1 dose (uncomplicated disease only) **AND**
- Erythromycin 50 mg/kg/day PO q6h, max 2gm/day x 7 days **OR**

-Azithromycin (Zithromax) 20 mg/kg PO x 1 dose, max 1 gm

Disseminated Gonococcal Infection:
-Ceftriaxone (Rocephin) 50 mg/kg/day (max 2gm/day) IV/IM q24h x 7 days
AND
-Azithromycin (Zithromax) 20 mg/kg (max 1gm) PO x 1 dose **OR**
-Erythromycin 40 mg/kg/day PO q6h (max 2gm/day) x 7 days **OR**
-Doxycycline 100 mg PO bid.

Gonorrhea in Children ≥ 45 kg and ≥8 years:
Uncomplicated Vulvovaginitis, Cervicitis, Urethritis, Proctitis, or Pharyngitis:
-Ceftriaxone (Rocephin) 125 mg IM x 1 dose **OR** cefixime (Suprax) 400 mg PO x 1 dose or ofloxacin (Floxin) 400 mg PO x 1 **dose**
     AND
-Azithromycin (Zithromax) 1000 mg PO x 1 dose **OR**
-Doxycycline 100 mg PO bid x 7 days.

Disseminated Gonococcal Infection:
-Ceftriaxone (Rocephin) 1000 mg/day IV/IM q24h x 7 days OR cefotaxime (Claforan) 1000 mg IV q8h x 7 days **AND**
-Azithromycin (Zithromax) 1000 mg PO x 1 dose **OR**
-Doxycycline 100mg PO bid x 7 days.

10. **Symptomatic Medications:**
     -Acetaminophen (Tylenol) 10-15 mg/kg/dose PO/PR q4-6h prn.
11. **Extras and X-rays:** Pelvic ultrasound; social services consult.
12. **Labs:** beta-HCG pregnancy test, CBC, SMA 7 and 12. GC culture and chlamydia test, RPR or VDRL. UA with micro; urine pregnancy test.

Pediculosis

Pediculosis Capitis (head lice):
-Permethrin (Nix) is the preferred treatment. Available in a 1% cream rinse that is applied to the scalp and hair for 10 minutes. A single treatment is adequate, but a second treatment may be applied 7-10 days after the first treatment [cream rinse: 1% 60 mL].
-Pyrethrin (Rid, A-2000, R&C). Available as a shampoo that is applied to the scalp and hair for 10 minutes. A repeat application 7-10 days later may sometimes be necessary [shampoo (0.3% pyrethrin, 3% piperonyl butoxide): 60, 120, 240 mL].
-For infestation of eyelashes, apply petrolatum ointment tid-qid for 8-10 days and mechanically remove the lice.

Pediculosis Corporis (body lice):
-Treatment consists of improving hygiene and cleaning clothes. Infested clothing should be washed and dried at hot temperatures to kill the lice.

Pediculicides are not necessary.

Pediculosis Pubis (pubic lice, "crabs"): Permethrin (Nix) or pyrethrin-based products may be used as described above for pediculosis capitis. Retreatment is recommended 7-10 days later.

Scabies

Treatment:

Bathe with soap and water; scrub and remove scaling or crusted detritus; towel dry. All clothing and bed linen contaminated within past 2 days should be washed in hot water for 20 min.

Permethrin (Elimite) - 5% cream: Adults and children: Massage cream into skin from head to soles of feet. Remove by washing after 8 to 14 hours. Treat infants on scalp, temple and forehead. One application is curative. [cream: 5% 60 gm]

Lindane (Kwell, Gamma benzene) - available as 1% cream or lotion: Use 1% lindane for adults and older children; not recommended in pregnancy, infants, or on excoriated skin. 1-2 treatments are effective. Massage a thin layer from neck to toes (including soles). In adults, 20-30 gm of cream or lotion is sufficient for 1 application. Bathe after 8 hours. May be repeated in one week if mites remain or if new lesions appear. Contraindicated in children <2 years of age. [lotion: 1% 60, 473 mL; shampoo:1%: 60, 473 mL].

Dermatophytoses

Diagnostic procedures:
  (1) KOH prep of scales and skin scrapings for hyphae.
  (2) Fungal cultures are used for uncertain cases.

Treat for at least 4 weeks.

Tinea corporis (ringworm), cruris (jock itch), pedis (athlete's foot):
  -Ketoconazole (Nizoral) cream qd [2%: 15, 30, 60 gm].
  -Clotrimazole (Lotrimin) cream bid [1%: 15, 30, 45 gm].
  -Miconazole (Micatin) cream bid [2%: 15, 30 gm].
  -Econazole (Spectazole) cream bid [1%: 15, 30, 85 gm].
  -Oxiconazole (Oxistat) cream or lotion qd-bid [1% cream: 15, 30, 60 gm; 1% lotion: 30 mL].
  -Sulconazole (Exelderm) cream or lotion qd-bid [1% cream: 15, 30, 60 gm; 1% lotion: 30 mL].
  -Naftifine (Naftin) cream or gel applied bid [1%: 15, 30 gm].
  -Terbinafine (Lamisil) cream or applied bid [1% cream: 15, 30 gm; 1% gel: 5, 15, 30 gm].

Tinea capitis:

-Griseofulvin Microsize (Grisactin, Grifulvin V) 15-20 mg/kg/day PO qd, max 1000 mg/day [caps: 125, 250 mg; susp: 125 mg/5 mL; tabs: 250, 500 mg]

-Griseofulvin Ultramicrosize (Fulvicin P/G, Grisactin Ultra, Gris-PEG) 5-10 mg/kg/day PO qd, max 750 mg/day [tabs: 125, 165, 250, 330 mg].

-Give griseofulvin with whole-milk or fatty foods to increase absorption. May require 4-6 weeks of therapy and should be continued for two weeks beyond clinical resolution.

Tinea Unguium (Fungal Nail Infection):

-Griseofulvin (see dosage above) is effective, but may require up to 4 months of therapy.

Tinea Versicolor:

-Cover body surface from face to knees with selenium sulfide 2.5% lotion or selenium sulfide 1% shampoo daily for 30 minutes for 1 week, then monthly x 3 to help prevent recurrences.

Bite Wounds

1. **Admit to:**
2. **Diagnosis:** Bite Wound.
3. **Condition:** Guarded.
4. **Vital signs:** Call MD if:
5. **Activity:**
6. **Nursing:** Cooling measures prn temp >38° C, age appropriate pain scale.
7. **Diet:**
8. **IV Fluids:** D5 NS at maintenance rate.
9. Special Medications:

-Initiate antimicrobial therapy for: moderate/severe bite wounds, especially if edema or crush injury is present; puncture wounds, especially if bone, tendon sheath, or joint penetration may have occurred; facial bites; hand and foot bites; genital area bites; wounds in immunocompromised or asplenic patients.

Dog Bites and Cat Bites:

Oral: amoxicillin/clavulanate

Oral, penicillin allergic: extended-spectrum cephalosporins or trimethoprim-sulfamethoxazole PLUS clindamycin

IV: ampicillin-sulbactam

IV, penicillin allergic: extended spectrum cephalosporins or trimethoprim-sulfamethoxazole PLUS clindamycin

Reptile Bites:

Oral: amoxicillin-clavulanate

Oral, penicillin allergic: extended-spectrum cephalosporins or trimethoprim-sulfamethoxazole PLUS clindamycin

IV: ampicillin-sulbactam PLUS gentamicin

IV, penicillin allergic: clindamycin PLUS gentamicin

Human Bites:

Oral: amoxicillin-clavulanate

Oral, penicillin allergic: trimethoprim-sulfamethoxazole PLUS clindamycin

IV: ampicillin-sulbactam

IV, penicillin allergic: extended-spectrum cephalosporins or trimethoprim-sulfamethoxazole PLUS clindamycin

Antibiotic Dosages:

-Amoxicillin/clavulanate (Augmentin)

40 mg/kg/day of amoxicillin PO tid, max 500 mg/dose

[elixir 125 mg/5 mL, 250 mg/5 mL; tabs: 250, 500 mg; tabs, chew: 125, 250 mg] **OR**

-Amoxicillin/clavulanate (Augmentin BID)

40 mg/kg/day PO bid, max 875 mg (amoxicillin)/dose

[susp: 200 mg/5 mL, 400 mg/5 mL; tab: 875 mg; tabs, chew: 200, 400 mg]

-Cefpodoxime (Vantin)

10 mg/kg/day PO bid, max 800 mg/day

[susp: 50 mg/5 mL, 100 mg/5 mL; tabs: 100, 200 mg] **OR**

-Cefprozil (Cefzil)

30 mg/kg/day PO bid, max 1 gm/day

[susp 125 mg/5 mL, 250 mg/5 mL; tabs: 250, 500 mg] **OR**

-Cefixime (Suprax)

8 mg/kg/day PO bid-qd, max 400 mg/day

[susp: 100 mg/5 mL; tabs: 200, 400 mg]

-Trimethoprim/sulfamethoxazole (Bactrim, Septra)

6-8 mg/kg/day of TMP PO/IV bid, max 320 mg TMP/day

[inj per mL: TMP 16 mg/SMX 80 mg; susp per 5 mL: TMP 40 mg/SMX 200 mg; tab DS: TMP 160 mg/SMX 800 mg; tab SS: TMP 80mg/SMX 400 mg]

-Clindamycin (Cleocin) 10-30 mg/kg/day PO q6-8h, max 1800 mg/day or 25-40 mg/kg/day IV/IM q6-8h, max 4.8 gm/day [cap: 75, 150, 300 mg; soln: 75 mg/5mL]

-Ampicillin-sulbactam (Unasyn) 100-200 mg/kg/day ampicillin IV/IM a6h, max 12 gm ampicillin/day

[1.5 gm (ampicillin 1 gm and sulbactam 0.5 gm; 3 gm (ampicillin 2 gm and sulbactam 1 gm)]

-Cefotaxime (Claforan) 100-150 mg/kg/day IV/IM q6-8h, max 12 gm/day

-Ceftriaxone (Rocephin) 50 mg/kg/day IV/IM qd, max 2 gm/day

-Gentamicin (Garamycin) (normal renal function):

<5 year (except neonates): 7.5 mg/kg/day IV/IM q8h.

5-10 year: 6.0 mg/kg/day IV/IM q8h.

>10 year: 5.0 mg/kg/day IV/IM q8h.

Additional Considerations:

-Sponge away visible dirt. Irrigate with a copious volume of sterile saline by high-pressure syringe irrigation. Débride any devitalized tissue.

-Tetanus immunization if not up-to-date.

-Assess risk of rabies from animal bites and risk of hepatitis and HIV from human bites.

10. **Symptomatic Medications:**

-Ibuprofen (Motrin) 5-10 mg/kg/dose PO q6-8h prn **OR**

-Acetaminophen (Tylenol) 15 mg/kg PO/PR q4h prn temp >38°C or pain.

11. **Extras and X-rays:** X-ray views of site of injury.

12. **Labs:** CBC, SMA 7, wound culture.

Lyme Disease

1. **Admit to:**
2. **Diagnosis:** Lyme disease.
3. **Condition:**
4. **Vital signs:** Call MD if:
5. **Activity:**
6. **Nursing:**
7. **Diet:**
8. **IV Fluids:** Isotonic fluids at maintenance rate.
9. **Special Medications:**

Early Localized Disease:

Age >8 years: doxycycline 100 mg PO bid x 14-21 days [caps: 50, 100 mg; susp: 25 mg/5mL; syrup: 50 mg/5mL; tabs 50, 100 mg]

All ages: amoxicillin 25-50 mg/kg/day PO bid (max 3 gm/day) x 14-21 days [caps: 250,500 mg; drops: 50 mg/mL; susp; 125 mg/5mL, 200 mg/5mL, 250 mg/5mL, 400 mg/5mL; tabs: 500, 875 mg; tabs, chew: 125, 200, 250, 400 mg]

Early Disseminated and Late Disease:

Multiple Erythema Migrans: Take same oral regimen as for early disease but for 21 days.

Isolated Facial Palsy: Take same oral regimen as for early disease but for 21-28 days.

Arthritis: Take same oral regimen as for early disease but for 28 days.

Persistent or Recurrent Arthritis:

-Ceftriaxone (Rocephin) 75-100 mg/kg/day IM/IV 12-24h (max 2 gm/dose) for 14-21 days **OR**

-Penicillin G 300,000 U/kg/day IV q4h (max 20 million units/day) x 14-21 days.

Carditis or Meningitis or Encephalitis:
    -Ceftriaxone (Rocephin) 75-100 mg/kg/day IM/IV q12-24h (max 2 gm/dose)
        for 14-21 days **OR**
    -Penicillin G 300,000 U/kg/day IV q4h (max 20 million units/day) x 14-21 days.
Lyme disease vaccine is available for children $\geq$15 years of age.

10. **Symptomatic Medications:**
    -Ibuprofen (Advil) 5-10 mg/kg/dose PO q6-8h prn temp >38° C **OR**
    -Acetaminophen (Tylenol) 15 mg/kg PO/PR q4h prn temp >38° C.

11. **Extras and X-rays:** CXR, MRI

12. Labs: IgM-specific antibody titer usually peaks between weeks 3 and 6 after the onset of infection. Enzyme immunoassay (EIA) is the most commonly used test for detection of antibodies. The Western immunoblot test is the most useful for corroborating a positive or equivocal EIA test.

Gastrointestinal Disorders

Gastroenteritis

1. **Admit to:**
2. **Diagnosis:** Acute Gastroenteritis.
3. **Condition:**
4. **Vital signs:** Call MD if:
5. **Activity:**
6. **Nursing:** Inputs and outputs, daily weights, urine specific gravity.
7. **Diet:** Rehydralyte, Pedialyte or soy formula (Isomil DF), bland diet.
8. **IV Fluids:** See Dehydration, page 107.
9. **Special Medications:**

Severe Gastroenteritis with Fever, Gross Blood and Neutrophils in Stool (E coli, Shigella, Salmonella):

-Ceftriaxone (Rocephin) 50-75 mg/kg/day IV/IM q 12-24h, max 4 gm/day **OR**
-Cefixime (Suprax) 8 mg/kg/day PO bid-qd, max 400 mg/day [susp: 100 mg/5 mL; tabs: 200, 400 mg] **OR**
-Trimethoprim/sulfamethoxazole (Bactrim, Septra) 10 mg of TMP component/kg/day PO bid x 5-7d, max 320 mg TMP/day [susp per 5 mL: TMP 40 mg/SMX 200 mg; tab DS: TMP 160 mg/SMX 800 mg; tab SS: TMP 80mg/SMX 400 mg].

Salmonella (treat infants and patients with septicemia):

-Ceftriaxone (Rocephin) 50-75 mg/kg/day IV/IM q12-24h, max 4 gm/day **OR**
-Cefixime (Suprax) 8 mg/kg/day PO bid-qd, max 400 mg/day [susp: 100 mg/5 mL; tabs: 200, 400 mg] **OR**
-Ampicillin 100-200 mg/kg/day IV q6h, max 12 gm/day or 50-100 mg/kg/day PO qid x 5-7d, max 4 gm/day [caps: 250, 500 mg; drops: 100 mg/mL; susp: 125 mg/5 mL, 250 mg/5 mL, 500 mg/5 mL] **OR**
-Trimethoprim/sulfamethoxazole (Bactrim, Septra) 10 mg TMP/kg/day PO bid x 5-7d, max 320 mg TMP/day [susp per 5 mL: TMP 40 mg/SMX 200 mg; tab DS: TMP 160 mg/SMX 800 mg; tab SS: TMP 80mg/SMX 400 mg] **OR**
-If >18 years: Ciprofloxacin (Cipro) 250-750 mg PO q12h or 200-400 mg IV q12h [inj: 200, 400 mg; susp: 100 mg/mL; tabs: 100, 250, 500, 750 mg]

Antibiotic Associated Diarrhea and Pseudomembranous Colitis (Clostridium difficile):

-Treat for 7-10 days.
-Metronidazole (Flagyl) 30 mg/kg/day PO/IV (PO preferred) q8h x 7 days, max 4 gm/day. [inj: 500 mg; tabs: 250, 500 mg; suspension] **OR**
-Vancomycin (Vancocin) 40 mg/kg/day PO qid x 7 days, max 2 gm/day [caps: 125, 250 mg; oral soln: 250 mg/5 mL, 500 mg/6 mL]. Vancomycin therapy

is reserved for patients who are allergic to metronidazole or who have not responded to metronidazole therapy.

10. **Extras and X-rays:** Upright abdomen.
11. **Labs:** SMA7, CBC; stool Wright stain for leukocytes, Rotazyme. Stool culture and sensitivity for enteric pathogens; C difficile toxin and culture, ova and parasites; occult blood. Urine specific gravity, UA, blood culture and sensitivity.

Specific Therapy for Gastroenteritis

Shigella Sonnei:
-Treat x 5 days. Oral therapy is acceptable except for seriously ill patients. Ciprofloxacin should be considered for resistant strains but is not recommended for use for persons younger than 18 years of age.
-Ampicillin (preferred over amoxicillin) 50-100 mg/kg/day PO q6h, max 3 gm/day [caps: 250, 500 mg; drops: 100 mg/mL; susp: 125 mg/5 mL, 250 mg/5 mL; 500 mg/5 mL] **OR**
-Trimethoprim/sulfamethoxazole (Bactrim, Septra) 10 mg TMP/kg/day PO/IV q12h x 5 days [inj per mL: TMP 16mg/SMX 80mg; susp per 5 mL: TMP 40 mg/SMX 200 mg; tab DS: TMP 160 mg/SMX 800 mg; tab SS: TMP 80mg/SMX 400 mg] **OR**
-Ampicillin 50-80 mg/kg/day PO q6h, max 4 gm/day; or 100 mg/kg/day IV/IM q6h for 5-7 days, max 12 gm/day [caps: 250, 500 mg; susp: 125 mg/5 mL, 250 mg/5 mL] **OR**
-Ceftriaxone (Rocephin) 50-75 mg/kg/day IV/IM q 12-24h, max 4 gm/day **OR**
-Cefixime (Suprax) 8 mg/kg/day PO bid-qd, max 400 mg/day [susp: 100 mg/5 mL; tabs: 200, 400 mg].

Yersinia (sepsis):
-Most isolates are resistant to first-generation cephalosporins and penicillins.
-Trimethoprim/sulfamethoxazole (Bactrim, Septra) 10 mg/kg/day TMP PO q12h x 5-7days [susp per 5 mL: TMP 40 mg/SMX 200 mg; tab DS: TMP 160 mg/SMX 800 mg; tab SS: TMP 80mg/SMX 400 mg].

Campylobacter jejuni:
-Erythromycin 40 mg/kg/day PO q6h x 5-7 days, max 2 gm/day
  Erythromycin ethylsuccinate (EryPed, EES)
    [susp: 200 mg/5 mL, 400 mg/5 mL; tab: 400 mg; tab, chew: 200 mg]
  Erythromycin base (E-Mycin, Ery-Tab, Eryc)
    [cap, DR: 250 mg; tabs: 250, 333, 500 mg] **OR**
-Azithromycin (Zithromax)
  10 mg/kg PO x 1 on day 1 (max 500 mg), followed by 5 mg/kg/day PO qd on days 2-5 (max 250 mg)
  [cap: 250 mg; susp: 100 mg/5mL, 200 mg/5mL; tabs: 250, 600 mg]

Enteropathogenic E coli (Travelers Diarrhea):
  -Trimethoprim/sulfamethoxazole (Bactrim, Septra) 10 mg/kg/day TMP PO/IV bid [inj per mL: TMP 16 mg/SMX 80 mg; susp per 5 mL: TMP 40 mg/SMX 200 mg; tab DS: TMP 160 mg/SMX 800 mg; tab SS: TMP 80mg/SMX 400 mg].
  -Patients older than 8 years old: Doxycycline (Vibramycin) 2-4 mg/kg/day PO q12-24h, max 200 mg/day [caps: 50, 100 mg; susp: 25 mg/5mL; syrup: 50 mg/5mL; tabs 50, 100 mg].

Enteroinvasive E coli:
  -Antibiotic selection should be based on susceptibility testing of the isolate. If systemic infection is suspected, parenteral antimicrobial therapy should be given.

Giardia Lamblia:
  -Metronidazole is the drug of choice. A 5-7 day course of therapy has a cure rate of 80-95%. Furazolidone is 72-100% effective when given for 7-10 days. Albendazole is also an acceptable alternative when given for 5 days.
  -Metronidazole (Flagyl) 15 mg/kg/day PO q8h x 5-7 days (max 4 gm/day) [tabs: 250, 500 mg; suspension] **OR**
  -Furazolidone (Furoxone) 5-8.8 mg/kg/day PO qid for 7-10 days, max 400 mg/day [susp: 50 mg/15 mL; tab: 100 mg] **OR**
  -Albendazole (Albenza): if > 2 years, 400 mg PO qd x 5 days [tab: 200mg; suspension]

Entamoeba Histolytica:
  Asymptomatic cyst carriers:
    -Iodoquinol (Yodoxin) 30-40 mg/kg/day PO q8h (max 1.95 gm/day) x 20 days [tabs: 210, 650 mg; powder for reconstitution] **OR**
    -Paromomycin (Humatin) 25-35 mg/kg/day PO q8h x 7 days [cap: 250 mg] **OR**
    -Diloxanide: 20 mg/kg/day PO q8h x 10 days, max 1500 mg/day. (Available only through CDC).
  Mild-to-moderate intestinal symptoms with no dysentery:
    -Metronidazole (Flagyl): 35-50 mg/kg/day PO q8h x 10 days, max 2250 mg/day [tabs: 250, 500 mg; suspension] followed by:
    -Iodoquinol (Yodoxin) 30-40 mg/kg/day PO q8h (max 1.95 gm/day) x 20 days [tabs: 210, 650 mg; powder for reconstitution] **OR**
    -Paromomycin (Humatin) 25-35 mg/kg/day PO q8h x 7 days [cap: 250 mg] **OR**
    -Diloxanide: 20 mg/kg/day PO q8h x 10 days, max 1500 mg/day. (Available only through CDC).
  Dysentery or extraintestinal disease (including liver abscess):
    -Metronidazole (Flagyl): 35-50 mg/kg/day PO q8h x 10 days, max 2250 mg/day [tabs: 250, 500 mg; suspension] followed by:
    -Iodoquinol (Yodoxin) 30-40 mg/kg/day PO q8h (max 1.95 gm/day) x 20 days [tabs: 210, 650 mg; powder for reconstitution] **OR**

-Paromomycin (Humatin) 25-35 mg/kg/day PO q8h x 7 days [cap: 250 mg]
OR
-Diloxanide: 20 mg/kg/day PO q8h x 10 days, max 1500 mg/day. (Available only through CDC).

Hepatitis A

1. **Admit to:**
2. **Diagnosis:** Hepatitis A.
3. **Condition:**
4. **Vital signs:** Call MD if:
5. **Activity:** Up ad lib.
6. **Nursing:** Contact precautions.
7. **Diet:**
8. **IV Fluids:** D5NS IV at maintenance rate.
9. **Symptomatic Medications:**
   -Trimethobenzamide (Tigan)
   15 mg/kg/day IM/PO/PR q6-8h, max 100 mg/dose if <13.6 kg or 200 mg/dose if 13.6-41kg.
   [caps: 100, 250 mg; inj: 100 mg/mL; supp: 100, 200 mg].
   -Acetaminophen (Tylenol) 15 mg/kg PO/PR q4h prn temp >38° C or pain.
   -Meperidine (Demerol) 1 mg/kg IV/IM q2-3h prn pain.
10. **Special Medications:**
   -Hepatitis A immune globulin, 0.02 mL/kg IM (usually requires multiple injections at different sites), when given within 2 weeks after exposure to HAV, is 85% effective in preventing symptomatic infection.
   -Hepatitis A vaccine (Havrix) if ≥2 years: 0.5 mL IM, repeat in 6-12 months.
11. **Extras and X-rays:** Abdominal x-ray series.
12. **Labs:** IgM anti-HAV antibody, HAV IgG, liver function tests, INR, PTT, stool culture for enteric pathogens.

Hepatitis B

1. **Admit to:**
2. **Diagnosis:** Hepatitis B.
3. **Condition:** Guarded.
4. **Vital signs:** Call MD if:
5. **Activity:**
6. **Nursing:** Standard precautions.
7. **Diet:** Low-fat diet
8. **IV Fluids:** Isotonic fluids at maintenance rate.

9. Symptomatic Medications:
-Trimethobenzamide (Tigan)

15 mg/kg/day IM/PO/PR q6-8h, max 100 mg/dose if <13.6 kg or 200 mg/dose if 13.6-41kg.

[caps: 100, 250 mg; inj: 100 mg/mL; supp: 100, 200 mg].

-Diphenhydramine (Benadryl) 1 mg/kg/dose IV/IM/IO/PO q6h prn pruritus or nausea, max 50 mg/dose **OR**

-Acetaminophen (Tylenol)15 mg/kg PO/PR q4h prn temp >38° C or pain.

-Meperidine (Demerol) 1 mg/kg IV/IM q2-3h prn pain.

Post exposure prophylaxis for previously unimmunized persons:
-Hepatitis B immune globulin 0.06 mL/kg (minimum 0.5 mL) IM x1 AND

-Hepatitis B vaccine 0.5 mL IM (complete three-dose series with second dose in one month and third dose in six months)

10. Extras and X-rays11. Labs:

-IgM anti-HAV, IgM anti-HBc, HBsAg, anti-HCV; alpha-1-antitrypsin, ANA, ferritin, ceruloplasmin, urine copper, liver function tests, INR, PTT.

Ulcerative Colitis

1. Admit to:

2. Diagnosis: Ulcerative colitis.

3. Condition:

4. Vital signs: Call MD if:

5. Activity:

6. Nursing: Daily weights, inputs and outputs.

7. Diet: NPO except for ice chips; no milk products.

8. IV Fluids:

9. Special Medications:
-Mesalamine (Asacol): 50 mg/kg/day PO q8-12h, max 800 mg PO TID [tab, EC: 400 mg] **OR**

-Mesalamine (Pentasa) 50 mg/kg/day PO q6-12h, max 1000 mg PO qid [cap, CR: 250 mg] **OR**

-Mesalamine (Rowasa) >12 years: 60 mL (4 gm) retention enema at bedtime retained overnight for approximately 8 hrs [4 gm/60 mL] OR > 12 years: mesalamine (Rowasa) 1 suppository PR bid [supp: 500 mg] **OR**

-Olsalazine sodium (Dipentum) >12 years: 500 mg PO with food bid [cap: 250 mg] **OR**

-Sulfasalazine (Azulfidine), children >2 years:

Mild exacerbation: 40-50 mg/kg/day PO q6h

Moderate to severe exacerbation: 50-75 mg/kg/day PO q4-6h, max 6 gm/day.

Maintenance therapy: 30-50 mg/kg/day PO q4-8h, max 2 gm/day.

[susp: 50 mg/mL; tab, EC: 500 mg] **OR**

-Hydrocortisone retention enema 100 mg PR qhs **OR**

-Hydrocortisone acetate 90 mg aerosol foam PR qd-bid or 25 mg supp PR bid.

-Prednisone 1-2 mg/kg/day PO qAM or bid (max 40-60 mg/day).

Other Medications:

-Vitamin B_{12} 100 mcg IM qd x 5 days, then 100-200 mcg IM q month.

-Multivitamin PO qAM or 1 ampule IV qAM.

-Folic acid 1 mg PO qd.

10. **Extras and X-rays:** Upright abdomen, GI consult.
11. **Labs:** CBC, platelets, SMA 7, Mg, ionized calcium; liver panel, blood culture and sensitivity x 2. Stool culture and sensitivity for enteric pathogens, ova and parasites, C. difficile toxin and culture, Wright's stain.

Parenteral Nutrition

1. **Admit to:**
2. **Diagnosis:**
3. **Condition:**
4. **Vital signs:** Call MD if:
5. **Nursing:** Daily weights, inputs and outputs; measure head circumference and height. Fingerstick glucose bid.
6. **Diet:**

Total Parenteral Nutrition:

-Calculate daily protein solution fluid requirement less fluid from lipid and other sources. Calculate total amino acid requirement.

-Protein: Neonates and infants start with 0.5 gm/kg/day and increase to 2-3 gm/kg/day. For children and young adults, start with 1 gm/kg/day, and increase by 1.0 gm/kg/day (max 2-3 gm/kg/day). Calculate percent amino acid to be infused: amino acid requirement in grams divided by the volume of fluid from the dextrose/protein solution in mL x 100.

-Advance daily dextrose concentration as tolerated, while following blood glucose levels. Usual maximum concentration is D35W.

Total Parenteral Nutrition Requirements			
	Infants-25 kg	25-45 kg	>45 kg
Calories	90-120 kcal/kg/day	60-105 kcal/kg/day	40-75 kcal/kg/day
Fluid	120-180 mL/kg/day	120-150 mL/kg/day	50-75 mL/kg/day
Dextrose	4-6 mg/kg/min	7-8 mg/kg/min	7-8 mg/kg/min

	Infants-25 kg	25-45 kg	>45 kg
Protein	2-3 gm/kg/day	1.5-2.5 gm/kg/day	0.8-2.0 gm/kg/day
Sodium	2-6 mEq/kg/day	2-6 mEq/kg/day	60-150 mEq/day
Potassium	2-5 mEq/kg/day	2-5 mEq/kg/day	70-150 mEq/day
Chloride	2-3 mEq/kg/day	2-3 mEq/kg/day	2-3 mEq/kg/day
Calcium	1-2 mEq/kg/day	1 mEq/kg/day	0.2-0.3 mEq/kg/day
Phosphate	0.5-1 mM/kg/day	0.5 mM/kg/day	7-10 mM/1000 cal
Magnesium	1-2 mEq/kg/day	1 mEq/kg/day	0.35-0.45 mEq/kg/day
Multi-Trace Element Formula	1 mL/day	1 mL/day	1 mL/day

Multivitamin (Peds MVI or MVC 9+3)	
<2.5 kg	2 mL/kg Peds MVI
2.5 kg -11 year	5 mL/day Peds MVI
≥11 years	MVC 9+3 10 mL/day

Dextrose Infusion:
-Dextrose mg/kg/min = [% dextrose x rate (mL/hr) x 0.167] ÷ kg
-Normal Starting Rate: 6-8 mg/kg/min

Lipid Solution:
-Minimum of 5% of total calories should be from fat emulsion. Max of 40% of calories as fat (10% soln = 1 gm/10 mL = 1.1 kcal/mL; 20% soln = 2 gm/10 mL = 2.0 kcal/mL). 20% Intralipid is preferred in most patients.
-For neonates, begin fat emulsion at 0.5 gm/kg/day and advance to 0.5-1 gm/kg/day.
-For infants, children and young adults, begin at 1 gm/kg/day, advance as tolerated by 0.5-1 gm/kg/day; max 3 gm/kg/day or 40% of calories/day.
-Neonates - infuse over 20-24h; children and infants - infuse over 16-24h, max 0.15 gm/kg/hr.
-Check serum triglyceride 6h after infusion (maintain <200 mg/dL)

Peripheral Parenteral Supplementation:
-Calculate daily fluid requirement less fluid from lipid and other sources.

Then calculate protein requirements: Begin with 1 gm/kg/day. Advance daily protein by 0.5-0.6 gm/kg/day to maximum of 3 gm/kg/day.

-Protein requirement in grams ÷ fluid requirement in mL x 100 = % amino acids.

-Begin with maximum tolerated dextrose concentration. (Dextrose concentration >12.5% requires a central line.)

-Calculate maximum fat emulsion intake (3 gm/kg/day), and calculate volume of 20% fat required (20 gm/100 mL = 20 %):

[weight (kg) x gm/kg/day] ÷ 20 x 100 = mL of 20% fat emulsion.

Start with 0.5-1.0 gm/kg/day lipid, and increase by 0.5-1.0 gm/kg/day until 3 gm/kg/day. Deliver over 18-24 hours.

-Draw blood 4-6h after end of infusion for triglyceride level.

7. **Extras and X-rays:** CXR, plain film for line placement, dietitian consult.

8. **Labs:**

Daily labs: Glucose, Na, K, Cl, HCO_3, BUN, creatinine, osmolarity, CBC, cholesterol, triglyceride, urine glucose and specific gravity.

Twice-weekly Labs: Calcium, phosphate, Mg, SMA-12.

Weekly Labs: Protein, albumin, prealbumin, Mg, direct and indirect bilirubin, AST, GGT, alkaline phosphatase, iron, TIBC, transferrin, retinol-binding protein, INR, PT/PTT, zinc, copper, B12, folate, 24h urine nitrogen and creatinine.

Gastroesophageal Reflux

A. **Treatment:**

-Thicken feedings; give small volume feedings; keep head of bed elevated 30 degrees.

-Metoclopramide (Reglan) 0.1-0.2 mg/kg/dose PO qid 20-30 minutes prior to feedings, max 1 mg/kg/day [concentrated soln: 10 mg/mL; syrup: 1 mg/mL; tab: 10 mg]

-Cimetidine (Tagamet) 20-40 mg/kg/day IV/PO q6h (20-30 min before feeding) [inj: 150 mg/mL; oral soln: 60 mg/mL; tabs: 200, 300, 400, 800 mg]

-Ranitidine (Zantac) 2-4 mg/kg/day IV q8h or 4-6 mg/kg/day PO q12h [inj: 25 mg/mL; liquid: 15 mg/mL; tabs: 75, 150, 300 mg]

-Erythromycin (prokinetic agent) 2-3 mg/kg/dose PO q6-8h. [ethylsuccinate susp: 200 mg/5mL, 400 mg/5mL] Concomitant cisapride is contraindicated due to potentially fatal drug interaction.

-Cisapride (Propulsid) 0.15-0.3 mg/kg/dose PO tid-qid [susp: 1 mg/mL; tab, scored: 10 mg]. Available via limited-access protocol only (Janssen, 1-800-Janssen) due to risk of serious cardiac arrhythmias.

B. **Extras and X-rays:** Upper GI series, pH probe, gastroesophageal nuclear scintigraphy (milk scan), endoscopy.

Constipation

I. Management of Constipation in Infants

A. Glycerin suppositories are effective up to 6 months of age: 1 suppository rectally prn. Barley malt extract, 1-2 teaspoons, can be added to a feeding two to three times daily. Four to six ounces prune juice is often effective. After 6 months of age, lactulose 1 to 2 mL/kg/day is useful.

B. Infants that do not respond may be treated with emulsified mineral oil (Haley's MO) 2 mL/kg/dose PO bid, increasing as needed to 6-8 oz per day.

II. Management of Constipation in Children >2 years of Age

A. The distal impaction should be removed with hypertonic phosphate enemas (Fleet enema). Usually three enemas are administered during a 36 to 48 hour period.

B. Lactulose may also be used at 5 to 10 mL PO bid, increasing as required up to 45 mL PO bid.

C. Emulsified mineral oil (Haley's MO) may be begun at 2 mL/kg/dose PO bid and increased as needed up to 6 to 8 oz per day.

D. Milk of magnesia: Preschoolers are begun at 2 tsp PO bid, with adjustments made to reach a goal of one to three substantial stools a day over 1 to 2 weeks. Older children: 1-3 tablets (311 mg magnesium hydroxide/chewable tablet) PO bid prn.

E. A bulk-type stool softener (eg, Metamucil) should be initiated. Increase intake of high-residue foods (eg fruits, vegetables), bran, and whole grain products. Water intake should be increased. Push oral fluids.

III. Stool Softeners and Laxatives:

A. Docusate sodium (Colace):

<3y	20-40 mg/day PO q6-24h
3-6y	20-60 mg/day PO q6-24h
6-12y	40-150 mg/day PO q6-24h
≥12y	50-400 mg/day PO q6-24h

[caps: 50,100, 250 mg; oral soln: 10 mg/mL, 50 mg/mL]

B. Magnesium hydroxide (Milk of Magnesia) 0.5 mL/kg/dose or 2-5 year: 5-15 mL; 6-12y: 15-30 mL; >12y: 30-60 mL PO prn.

C. Hyperosmotic soln (CoLyte or GoLytely) 15-20 mL/kg/hr PO/NG.

D. Polyethylene glycol (MiraLax)

3-6 year: 1 tsp powder dissolved in 3 ounces fluid PO qd-tid

6-12 year: 1/2 tablespoon powder dissolved in 4 ounces fluid PO qd-tid

≥12 year: one tablespoon powder dissolved in 8 ounces fluid PO qd-tid

E. Senna (Senokot, Senna-Gen) 10-20 mg/kg PO/PR qhs prn (max 872 mg/day) [granules: 362 mg/teaspoon; supp: 652 mg; syrup: 218 mg/5mL; tabs: 187, 217, 600 mg]

    F. Sennosides (Agoral, Senokot, Senna-Gen), 2-6 years: 3-8.6 mg/dose PO qd-bid; 6-12 years: 7.15-15 mg/dose PO qd-bid; > 12 years: 12-25 mg/dose PO qd-bid [granules per 5 mL: 8.3, 15, 20 mg; liquid: 33 mg/mL; syrup: 8.8 mg/5 mL; tabs: 6, 8.6, 15, 17, 25 mg]

IV. **Diagnostic Evaluation:** Anorectal manometry, anteroposterior and lateral abdominal radiographs, lower GI study of unprepared colon.

Toxicology

Poisonings

Gastric Decontamination:

Ipecac Syrup:

<6 months: not recommended

6-12 months: 5-10 mL PO followed by 10-20 mL/kg of water

1-12 years: 15 mL PO followed by 10-20 mL/kg of water

>12 years: 30 mL PO followed by 240 mL of water

May repeat dose one time if vomiting does not occur within 20-30 minutes. Syrup of ipecac is contraindicated in corrosive or hydrocarbon ingestions or in patients without a gag reflex.

Activated Charcoal: 1 gm/kg/dose (max 50 gm) PO/NG; the first dose should be given using product containing sorbitol as a cathartic. Repeat 1/2 of initial dose q4h.

Gastric Lavage: Left side down, with head slightly lower than body; place large-bore orogastric tube and check position by injecting air and auscultating. Normal saline lavage: 15 mL/kg boluses until clear (max 400 mL), then give activated charcoal or other antidote. Save initial aspirate for toxicological exam. Gastric lavage is contraindicated if corrosives, hydrocarbons, or sharp objects were ingested.

Cathartics:

-Magnesium citrate 6% soln:

<6 years: 2-4 mL/kg/dose PO/NG

6-12 years: 100-150 mL PO/NG

>12 years: 150-300 mL PO/NG

Antidotes to Common Poisonings

Narcotic or Propoxyphene Overdose:

-Naloxone (Narcan) 0.1 mg/kg/dose (max 4 mg) IV/IO/ET/IM, may repeat q2min.

Methanol or Ethylene Glycol Overdose:

-Ethanol 8-10 mL/kg (10% inj soln) IV in D5W over 30min, then 0.8-1.4 mL/kg/hr. Maintain ethanol level at 100-130 mg/dL.

Carbon Monoxide Inhalation:

-Oxygen 100% or hyperbaric oxygen.

Cyanide Ingestion:

-Amyl nitrite; break ampule and inhale ampule contents for 30 seconds q1min until sodium nitrite is administered. Use new amp q3min **AND**

-Sodium nitrite 0.33 mL/kg of 3% inj soln (max 10 mL) IV over 5 minutes. Repeat 1/2 dose 30 min later if inadequate clinical response.

Followed By:

-Sodium thiosulfate 1.65 mL/kg of 25% soln (max 50 mL) IV.

Phenothiazine Reaction (Extrapyramidal Reaction):

-Diphenhydramine (Benadryl) 1 mg/kg IV/IM q6h x 4 doses (max 50 mg/dose) followed by 5 mg/kg/day PO q6h for 2-3 days.

Digoxin Overdose:

-Digibind (Digoxin immune Fab). Dose (# vials) = digoxin level in ng/mL x body wt (kg)/100 **OR**

Dose (# of vials) = mg of digoxin ingested divided by 0.6

Benzodiazepine Overdose:

-Flumazenil (Romazicon) 0.01 mg/kg IV (max 0.5 mg). Repeat dose if symptoms return.

Alcohol Overdose: Cardiorespiratory support

-**Labs:** Blood glucose; CBC, ABG, rapid toxicology screen.

-Treatment: Dextrose 0.5-1 gm/kg (2-4 mL/kg D25W or 5-10 mL/kg D10W), max 25 gm.

-Naloxone (Narcan) 0.1 mg/kg (max 2 mg) IV, repeat q2min prn to max dose 8-10 mg if drug overdose suspected. For extreme agitation, give diazepam 0.1-0.5 mg/kg IV (max 5 mg if < 5 years, 10 mg if ≥5 years).

Organophosphate Toxicity

-Atropine: 0.01-0.02 mg/kg/dose (minimum dose 0.1mg, maximum dose 0.5 mg in children and 1 mg in adolescents) IM/IV/SC. May repeat prn.

-Pralidoxime (2-PAM): 20-50 mg/kg/dose IM/IV. Repeat in 1-2 hrs if muscle weakness has not been relieved, then at 10-12 hr intervals if cholinergic signs recur.

Anticholinergic Toxicity

-Physostigmine (Antilirium): 0.01-0.03 mg/kg/dose IV; may repeat after 15-20 minutes to a maximum total dose of 2 mg.

Heparin Overdose

-Protamine sulfate dosage is determined by the most recent dosage of heparin and the time elapsed since the overdose.

Dosage of Protamine Sulfate	
Time Elapsed	**IV Dose of Protamine (mg) to Neutralize 100 units of Heparin**
Immediate	1-1.5
30-60 minutes	0.5-0.75

Time Elapsed	IV Dose of Protamine (mg) to Neutralize 100 units of Heparin
> 2 hrs	0.25-0.375

Warfarin Overdose
  -Phytonadione (Vitamin K_1)
  -If no bleeding and rapid reversal needed and patient will require further oral anticoagulation therapy, give 0.5-2 mg IV/SC
  -If no bleeding and rapid reversal needed and patient will **not** require further oral anticoagulation therapy, give 2-5 mg IV/SC
  -If significant bleeding but not life-threatening, give 0.5-2 mg IV/SC
  -If significant bleeding and life-threatening, give 5 mg IV [inj: 2 mg/mL, 10 mg/mL] or give fresh frozen plasma (FFP) 10-15 ml/kg.

Acetaminophen Overdose

1. **Admit to:**
2. **Diagnosis:** Acetaminophen overdose.
3. **Condition:**
4. **Vital signs:** Call MD if
5. **Nursing:** ECG monitoring, inputs and outputs, pulse oximeter, aspiration precautions.
6. **Diet:**
7. **IV Fluids:**
8. **Special Medications:**
   -Gastric lavage with 10 mL/kg (if >5 years, use 150-200 mL) of normal saline by nasogastric tube if <60 minutes after ingestion.
   -Activated charcoal (if recent ingestion) 1 gm/kg PO/NG q2-4h, remove via suction prior to acetylcysteine.
   -N-Acetylcysteine (Mucomyst, NAC) loading dose 140 mg/kg PO/NG, then 70 mg/kg PO/NG q4h x 17 doses (20% soln diluted 1:4 in carbonated beverage); follow acetaminophen levels. Continue for full treatment course even if serum levels fall below nomogram.
   -Phytonadione (Vitamin K) 1-5 mg PO/IV/IM/SQ (if INR >1.5).
   -Fresh frozen plasma should be administered if INR >3. 10-15 ml/kg.
9. **Extras and X-rays:** Portable CXR. Nephrology consult for charcoal hemoperfusion.
10. **Labs:** CBC, SMA 7, liver panel, amylase, INR/PTT; SGOT, SGPT, bilirubin, acetaminophen level now and q4h until nondetectable. Plot serum acetaminophen level on Rumack-Matthew nomogram to assess severity of

ingestion unless sustained-release Tylenol was ingested. Toxicity is likely with ingestion $\geq$150 mg/kg (or 7.5 gm in adolescents/adults).

Lead Toxicity

1. **Admit to:**
2. **Diagnosis:** Lead toxicity.
3. **Condition:**
4. **Vital signs:** Call MD if
5. **Nursing:** ECG monitoring, inputs and outputs, pulse oximeter.
6. **Diet:**
7. **IV Fluids:**
8. **Special Medications:**

Symptoms of lead encephalopathy and/or blood level >70 mcg/DL:
-Treat for five days with edetate calcium disodium and dimercaprol:
-Edetate calcium disodium 250 mg/m^2/dose IM q4h or 50 mg/kg/day continuous IV infusion or 1-1.5 gm/m^2 IV as either an 8- or 24-hr infusion.
-Dimercaprol (BAL): 4 mg/kg/dose IM q4h

Symptomatic lead poisoning without encephalopathy or asymptomatic with blood level >70 mcg/dL:
-Treat for 3–5 days with edetate calcium disodium and dimercaprol until blood lead level <50 mcg/dL.
-Edetate calcium disodium 167 mg/m^2 IM q4h or 1 gm/m^2 as a 8- to 24-hr continuous IV infusion.
-Dimercaprol (BAL): 4 mg/kg IM x 1 then 3 mg/kg/dose IM q4h.

Asymptomatic children with blood lead level 45-69 mcg/dL:
-Edetate calcium disodium 25 mg/kg/day as a 8-24 hr IV infusion or IV q12h
OR
-Succimer (Chemet): 10 mg/kg/dose (or 350 mg/m^2/dose) PO q8h x 5 days, followed by 10 mg/kg/dose (or 350 mg/m^2/dose) PO q12h x 14 days [cap: 100 mg].

9. **Labs:** CBC, SMA 7, blood lead level, serum iron level.

Theophylline Overdose

1. **Admit to:**
2. **Diagnosis:** Theophylline overdose.
3. **Condition:**
4. **Vital signs:** Call MD if:
5. **Activity:**
6. **Nursing:** ECG monitoring until serum level is less than 20 mcg/mL; inputs

and outputs, aspiration and seizure precautions.

7. **Diet:**

8. **IV Fluids:** Give IV fluids at rate to treat dehydration.

9. **Special Medications:**
   -No specific antidote is available.
   -Activated charcoal 1 gm/kg PO/NG (max 50 gm) q2-4h, followed by cathartic, regardless of time of ingestion. Repeat until theophylline level <20 mcg/mL.
   -Gastric lavage if greater than 20 mg/kg was ingested or if unknown amount ingested or if symptomatic.
   -Charcoal hemoperfusion if serum level >60 mcg/mL or signs of neurotoxicity, seizure, coma.

10. **Extras and X-rays:** Portable CXR, ECG.

11. **Labs:** CBC, SMA 7, theophylline level; INR/PTT, liver panel. Monitor K, Mg, phosphorus, calcium, acid/base balance.

Iron Overdose

1. **Admit to:**

2. **Diagnosis:** Iron overdose

3. **Condition:**

4. **Vital signs:** Call MD if:

5. **Activity:**

6. **Nursing:** Inputs and outputs.

7. **Diet:**

8. **IV Fluids:** Maintenance IV fluids.

9. **Special Medications:**
   Toxicity likely if >60 mg/kg elemental iron ingested.
   Possibly toxic if 20-60 mg/kg elemental iron ingested.
   Induce emesis with ipecac if recent ingestion (<1 hour ago). Charcoal is not effective. Gastric lavage if greater than 20 mg/kg of elemental iron ingested or if unknown amount ingested.
   If hypotensive, give IV fluids (10-20 mL/kg normal saline) and place the patient in Trendelenburg's position.
   Maintain urine output of >2 mL/kg/h.
   If peak serum iron is greater than 350 mcg/dL or if symptomatic, begin chelation therapy.
   -Deferoxamine (Desferal) 15 mg/kg/hr continuous IV infusion. Continue until metabolic acidosis has resolved, the patient is asymptomatic and has an iron level less than 150 mcg/dL.
   Exchange transfusion is recommended in severely symptomatic patients with serum iron >1,000 mcg/dL.

10. **Extras and X-rays:** KUB to determine if tablets are present in intestine.
11. **Labs:** Type and cross, CBC, electrolytes, serum iron, TIBC, INR/PTT, blood glucose, liver function tests, calcium.

Neurologic and Endocrinologic Disorders

Seizure and Status Epilepticus

1. **Admit to:** Pediatric intensive care unit.
2. **Diagnosis:** Seizure.
3. **Condition:**
4. **Vital signs:** Vitals and neurochecks q2-6h; call MD if:
5. **Activity:**
6. **Nursing:** Seizure and aspiration precautions, ECG and EEG monitoring.
7. **Diet:** NPO.
8. **IV Fluids:**
9. **Special Medications:**

Febrile Seizures: Control fever with antipyretics and cooling measures. Anticonvulsive therapy is usually not required.

Status Epilepticus:

1. Maintain airway, 100% O_2 by mask; obtain brief history, fingerstick glucose.
2. Start IV NS. If hypoglycemic, give 1-2 mL/kg D25W IV/IO (0.25-0.5 gm/kg).
3. Lorazepam (Ativan) 0.1 mg/kg (max 4 mg) IV/IM. Repeat q15-20 min x 3 prn.
4. Phenytoin (Dilantin) 15-18 mg/kg in normal saline at <1 mg/kg/min (max 50 mg/min) IV/IO. Monitor BP and ECG (QT interval).
5. If seizures continue, intubate and give phenobarbital loading dose of 15-20 mg/kg IV or 5 mg/kg IV every 15 minutes until seizures are controlled or 30 mg/kg is reached.
6. If seizures are refractory, consider midazolam (Versed) infusion (0.1 mg/kg/hr) or general anesthesia with EEG monitoring.
7. Rectal Valium gel formulation

   <2 years: not recommended

   2-5 years: 0.5 mg/kg

   6-11 years: 0.3 mg/kg

   ≥12 years: 0.2 mg/kg

   Round dose to 2.5, 5, 10, 15, and 20 mg/dose. Dose may be repeated in 4-12 hrs if needed. Do not use more than five times per month or more than once every five days.[rectal gel (Diastat): pediatric rectal tip - 5 mg/mL (2.5, 5, 10 mg size); adult rectal tip - 5 mg/mL (10, 15, 20 mg size)]

Generalized Seizures Maintenance Therapy:

-Carbamazepine (Tegretol):

<6 year: initially 10-20 mg/kg/day PO bid, then may increase in 5-7 day intervals by 5 mg/kg/day; usual max dose 35 mg/kg/day PO q6-8h.

6-12 year: initially 100 mg PO bid (10 mg/kg/day PO bid), then may increase by 100 mg/day at weekly intervals; usual maintenance dose 400-800 mg/day PO bid-qid.

>12 year: initially 200 mg PO bid, then may increase by 200 mg/day at weekly intervals; usual maintenance dose 800-1200 mg/day PO bid-tid. Dosing interval depends on product selected. Susp: q6-8h; tab: q8- 12h; tab, chew: q8-12h; tab, ER: q12h

[susp: 100 mg/5 mL; tab: 200 mg; tab, chewable: 100 mg; tab, ER: 100, 200, 400 mg] **OR**

-Divalproex sodium (Depakote, Valproic acid) PO: Initially 10-15 mg/kg/day bid-tid, then increase by 5-10 mg/kg/day weekly as needed; usual maintenance dose 30-60 mg/kg/day bid-tid. Up to 100 mg/kg/day tid-qid may be required if other enzyme-inducing anticonvulsants are used concomitantly. IV: total daily dose is equivalent to total daily oral dose but divide q6h. PR: dilute syrup 1:1 with water for use as a retention enema, loading dose 17-20 mg/kg x 1 or maintenance 10-15 mg/kg/dose q8h.

[cap: 250 mg; cap, sprinkle: 125 mg; inj: 100 mg/mL; syrup: 250 mg/5 mL; tab, DR: 125, 250, 500 mg] **OR**

-Phenobarbital (Luminal): Loading dose 10-20 mg/kg IV/IM/PO, then maintenance dose 3-5 mg/kg/day PO qd-bid.

[cap: 16 mg; elixir: 15 mg/5mL, 4 mg/mL; inj: 30 mg/mL, 60 mg/mL, 65 mg/mL, 130 mg/mL; tabs: 8, 15, 16, 30, 32, 60, 65,100 mg] **OR**

-Phenytoin (Dilantin): Loading dose 15-18 mg/kg IV/PO, then maintenance dose 5-7 mg/kg/day PO/IV q8-24h (only sustained release capsules may be dosed q24h).

[caps: 30, 100 mg; elixir: 125 mg/5 mL; inj: 50 mg/mL; tab, chewable: 50 mg]

-Fosphenytoin (Cerebyx): >5 years: loading dose 10-20 mg PE IV/IM, maintenance dose 4-6 mg/kg/day PE IV/IM q12-24h. Fosphenytoin 1.5 mg is equivalent to phenytoin 1 mg which is equivalent to fosphenytoin 1 mg phenytoin equivalent (PE) unit. Fosphenytoin is a water-soluble pro-drug of phenytoin and must be ordered as mg of phenytoin equivalent.

[inj: 150 mg (equivalent to phenytoin sodium 100 mg) in 2 mL vial; 750 mg (equivalent to phenytoin sodium 500 mg) in 10 mL vial]

Partial Seizures and Secondary Generalized Seizures:

-Carbamazepine (Tegretol), see above **OR**

-Phenytoin (Dilantin), see above.

-Phenobarbital (Luminal), see above **OR**

-Valproic acid (Depacon, Depakote, Depakene), see above.

-Lamotrigine (Lamictal):

    Adding to regimen containing valproic acid: 2-12 years: 0.15 mg/kg/day PO qd-bid during weeks 1-2, then increase to 0.3 mg/kg/day PO qd-bid during weeks 3-4, then increase q1-2 weeks by 0.3 mg/kg/day to maintenance dose 1-5 mg/kg/day (max 200 mg/day).

    >12 years: 25 mg PO qOD during weeks 1-2, then increase to 25 mg PO qd during weeks 3-4, then increase q1-2 weeks by 25-50 mg/day to maintenance dose of 100-400 mg/day PO qd-bid.

    Adding to regimen without valproic acid: 2-12 years: 0.6 mg/kg/day PO bid during weeks 1-2, then increase to 1.2 mg/kg/day PO bid during weeks 3-4, then increase q1-2 weeks by 1.2 mg/kg/day to maintenance dose 5-15 mg/kg/day PO bid (max 400 mg/day).

    >12 years: 50 mg PO qd weeks 1-2, then increase to 50 mg PO bid during weeks 3-4, then increase q1-2 weeks by 100 mg/day to maintenance dose 300-500 mg/day PO bid.

    [tabs: 25, 100, 150, 200 mg].

-Primidone (Mysoline) PO: 8 years: 50-125 mg/day qhs, increase by 50-125 mg/day q3-7d; usual dose 10-25 mg/kg/day tid-qid.

    $\geq$8 years: 125-250 mg qhs; increase by 125-250 mg/day q3-7d, usual dose 750-1500 mg/day tid-qid (max 2 gm/day).

    [susp: 250 mg/5mL; tabs: 50, 250 mg]

10. **Extras and X-rays:** MRI with and without gadolinium, EEG with hyperventilation, CXR, ECG. Neurology consultation.

11. **Labs:** ABG/CBG, CBC, SMA 7, calcium, phosphate, magnesium, liver panel, VDRL, anticonvulsant levels, blood and urine culture. UA, drug and toxin screen.

Therapeutic Serum Levels	
Carbamazepine	4-12 mcg/mL
Clonazepam	20-80 ng/mL
Ethosuximide	40-100 mcg/mL
Phenobarbital	15-40 mcg/mL
Phenytoin	10-20 mcg/mL
Primidone	5-12 mcg/mL
Valproic acid	50-100 mcg/mL

Adjunctive Anticonvulsants

Felbamate (Felbatol)

2-14 years: 15 mg/kg/day PO tid-qid, increase weekly by 15 mg/kg/day if needed to maximum of 45 mg/kg/day or 3600 mg/day (whichever is smaller).

≥14 years: 1200 mg/day PO tid-qid, increase weekly by 1200 mg/day if needed to maximum of 3600 mg/day

[susp: 600 mg/5 mL; tabs: 400, 600 mg]

Warning: due to risk of aplastic anemia and hepatic failure reported with this drug, written informed consent must be obtained from patient/parent prior to initiating therapy. Patients must have CBC, liver enzymes, and bilirubin monitored before starting drug therapy and q1-2 weeks during therapy. Discontinue the drug immediately if bone marrow suppression or elevated liver function tests occur.

Gabapentin (Neurontin)

2-12 years: 5-35 mg/kg/day PO q8h.

>12 years: initially 300 mg PO tid, titrate dose upward if needed; usual dose 900-1800 mg/day, maximum 3600 mg/day.

[caps: 100, 300, 400 mg; soln: 250 mg/5 mL; tabs: 600, 800 mg].

Adjunctive treatment of partial and secondarily generalized seizures.

Levetiracetam (Keppra)

≥16 years: 500 mg PO bid, may increase by 1000 mg/day q2 weeks to maximum of 3000 mg/day [tabs: 250, 500, 750 mg].

Tiagabine (Gabitril)

<12 years: dosing guidelines not established.

12-18 years: 4 mg PO qd x 1 week, then 4 mg bid x 1 week, then increase weekly by 4-8 mg/day and titrate to response; maximum dose 32 mg/day bid-qid [tabs: 2, 4, 12, 16, 20 mg]. Lower doses may be effective in patients not receiving enzyme-inducing drugs.

Topiramate (Topamax)

2-16 years with partial onset seizures: 1-3 mg/kg/day PO qhs x 1 week (max 25 mg/day), may increase q1-2 weeks by 1-3 mg/kg/day bid to usual maintenance dose 5-9 mg/kg/day bid.

2-16 years with primary generalized tonic clonic seizures: use slower initial titration rate to max of 6 mg/kg/day PO by the end of eight weeks.

>16 years with partial onset seizures: 50 mg/day qhs x 1 week, then 100 mg/day bid x 1 week, then increase by 50 mg/day q week; usual maintenance dose 200 mg bid, max 1600 mg/day.

>16 years with generalized tonic clonic seizures: use slower initial titration rate to usual maintenance dose 200 mg bid, max 1600 mg/day.

[caps, sprinkles: 15, 25, 50 mg; tabs: 25, 100, 200 mg].

Vigabatrin (Sabril) PO

3-9 years: 500 mg bid

>9 years: 1000 mg bid, may increase if needed to max 4000 mg/day.

[tab: 500 mg]. Most effective in complex partial seizures, with or without generalization. Should be used as add-on therapy in patients with drug-resistant seizures, not as monotherapy. Do not abruptly discontinue therapy; gradually taper to avoid rebound increase in seizure frequency and possible psychotic episodes.

Spasticity

1. **Admit to:**
2. **Diagnosis:** Cerebral palsy, spasticity.
3. **Condition:**
4. **Vital signs:**
5. **Activity:** Physical Therapy.
6. **Nursing:** Inputs and outputs; daily weights.
7. **Diet:** Regular.
8. **IV Fluids:** Isotonic fluids at maintenance rate if NPO.
9. **Special Medications:**
   -Baclofen (Lioresal)
      2-7 years: 10-15 mg/day PO q8h, titrate dose upwards by 5-15 mg/day q3 days to a maximum of 40 mg/day.
      >7 years: 10-15 mg/day PO q8h, titrate dose upwards by 5-15 mg/day q3 days to a maximum of 60 mg/day.
      [tabs: 10, 20 mg; suspension].
   -Diazepam (Valium), 0.12-0.8 mg/kg/day PO q6-8h or 0.04-0.3 mg/kg/dose IV/IM q4h prn.
      [inj: 5 mg/mL; soln: 1 mg/mL, 5 mg/mL; tabs: 2, 5, 10 mg].
   -Dantrolene (Dantrium), 0.5 mg/kg/dose PO bid, may increase q4-7 days by 0.5 mg/kg/day to maximum of 3 mg/kg/dose PO bid-qid up to 400 mg/day [caps: 25, 50, 100 mg; suspension].
10. **Extras and X-rays:** Occupational therapy consult; physical therapy consult; rehab consult.

New Onset Diabetes

1. **Admit to:**
2. **Diagnosis:** New Onset Diabetes Mellitus.
3. **Condition:**
4. **Vital signs:** Call MD if:
5. **Activity:** Up ad lib.
6. **Nursing:** Record labs on a flow sheet. Fingerstick glucose at 0700, 1200, 1700, 2100, 0200; diabetic and dietetic teaching.

7. **Diet:** Diabetic diet with 1000 kcal + 100 kcal/year of age. 3 meals and 3 snacks (between each meal and qhs.)
8. **IV Fluids:** Hep-lock with flush q shift.
9. **Special Medications:**
   -Goal is preprandial glucose of 100-200 mg/dL

Total Daily Insulin Dosage		
<5 Years (U/kg)	5-11 Years (U/kg)	12-18 Years (U/kg)
0.6-0.8	0.75-0.9	0.8-1.5

   -Divide 2/3 before breakfast and 1/3 before dinner. Give 2/3 of total insulin requirement as NPH and give 1/3 as lispro or regular insulin.
10. **Extras and X-rays:** CXR. Endocrine and dietary consult.
11. **Labs:** CBC, ketones; SMA 7 and 12, antithyroglobulin, antithyroid microsomal, anti-insulin, anti-islet cell antibodies. UA, urine culture and sensitivity; pregnancy test; urine ketones.

Diabetic Ketoacidosis

1. **Admit to:** Pediatric intensive care unit.
2. **Diagnosis:** Diabetic ketoacidosis.
3. **Condition:** Critical.
4. **Vital signs:** Call MD if:
5. **Activity:**
6. **Nursing:** ECG monitoring; capillary glucose checks q1-2h until glucose level is <200 mg/dL, daily weights, inputs and outputs. O_2 at 2-4 L/min by NC. Record labs on flow sheet.
7. **Diet:** NPO
8. **IV Fluids:** 0.9% saline 10-20 mL/kg over 1h, then repeat until blood pressure and pulse are normal. Then give 0.45% saline, and replace 1/2 of calculated deficit plus insensible loss over 8h, replace remaining 1/2 of deficit plus insensible losses over 16-24h. Keep urine output >1.0 mL/kg/hour.
   Add KCL when potassium is <6.0 mEq/dL

Serum K+	Infusate KCL
<3	40-60 mEq/L
3-4	30
4-5	20
5-6	10
>6	0

   Rate: 0.25-1 mEq KCL/kg/hr, maximum 1 mEq/kg/h or 20 mEq/h.

9. **Special Medications:**
   -Regular insulin(Humulin) 0.05-0.1 U/kg/hr (50 U in 500 mL NS) continuous IV infusion. Adjust to decrease glucose by 50-100 mg/dL/hr.
   -If glucose decreases at less than 50 mg/dL/hr, increase insulin to 0.14-0.2 U/kg/hr. If glucose decreases faster than 100 mg/dL/hr, continue insulin at 0.05-0.1 U/kg/h and add D5W to IV fluids.
   -When glucose approaches 250-300 mg/dL, add D5W to IV. Change to subcutaneous insulin (lispro or regular) when bicarbonate is >15, and patient is tolerating PO food; do not discontinue insulin drip until one hour after subcutaneous dose of insulin.
10. **Extras and X-rays:** Portable CXR, ECG. Endocrine and dietary consultation.
11. **Labs:** Dextrostixs q1-2h until glucose <200 mg/dL, then q4-6h. Glucose, potassium, phosphate, bicarbonate q3-4h; serum acetone, CBC. UA, urine ketones, culture and sensitivity.

Hematologic and Inflammatory Disorders

Sickle Cell Crisis

1. **Admit to:**
2. **Diagnosis:** Sickle Cell Anemia, Sickle Cell Crisis.
3. **Condition:**
4. **Vital signs:** Call MD if
5. **Activity:**
6. **Nursing:** Age appropriate pain scale.
7. **Diet:**
8. **IV Fluids:** D5 1/2 NS at 1.5-2.0 x maintenance.
9. **Special Medications:**
   -Oxygen 2-4 L/min by NC.
   -Morphine sulfate 0.1 mg/kg/dose (max 10-15 mg) IV/IM/SC q2-4h prn or
     follow bolus with infusion of 0.05-0.1 mg/kg/hr prn or 0.3-0.5 mg/kg PO q4h
     prn **OR**
   -Acetaminophen/codeine 0.5-1 mg/kg/dose (max 60 mg/dose) of codeine PO
     q4-6h prn [elixir: 12 mg codeine/5 mL; tabs: 15, 30, 60 mg codeine
     component] **OR**
   -Acetaminophen and hydrocodone [elixir per 5 mL: hydrocodone 2.5 mg,
     acetaminophen] 167 mg; tabs:
     Hydrocodone 2.5 mg, acetaminophen 500 mg;
     Hydrocodone 5 mg, acetaminophen 500 mg;
     Hydrocodone 7.5 mg, acetaminophen 500 mg,
     Hydrocodone 7.5 mg, acetaminophen 650 mg,
     Hydrocodone 10 mg, acetaminophen 500 mg,
     Hydrocodone 10 mg, acetaminophen 650 mg
     Children: 0.6 mg hydrocodone/kg/day PO q6-8h prn
     <2 year: do not exceed 1.25 mg/dose
     2-12 year: do not exceed 5 mg/dose
     >12 year: do not exceed 10 mg/dose

Patient-Controlled Analgesia
   -Morphine
     Basal rate 0.01-0.02 mg/kg/hr.
     Intermittent bolus dose 0.01-0.03 mg/kg.
     Bolus frequency ("lockout interval") every 6-15 minutes.
   -Hydromorphone (Dilaudid)
     Basal rate 0.0015-0.003 mg/kg/hr.
     Intermittent bolus dose 0.0015-0.0045 mg/kg.

Bolus frequency ("lockout interval") every 6-15 min

Adjunctive Therapy:

-Hydroxyzine (Vistaril) 0.5-1 mg/kg/dose PO q6h (max 50 mg/dose)

-Ibuprofen (Motrin) 10 mg/kg/dose PO q6h (max 800 mg/dose) **OR**

-Ketorolac (Toradol) 0.4 mg/kg/dose IV/IM q6h (max 30 mg/dose); maximum 3 days, then switch to oral ibuprofen

Maintenance Therapy:

-Hydroxyurea (Hydrea): 15 mg/kg/day PO qd, may increase by 5 mg/kg/day q12 weeks to a maximum dose of 35 mg/kg/day. Monitor for myelotoxicity. [caps: 200, 300, 400, 500 mg].

-Folic acid 1 mg PO qd (if >1 year).

-Transfuse PRBC 5 mL/kg over 2h, then 10 mL/kg over 2h, then check hemoglobin. If hemoglobin is less than 6-8 gm/dL, give additional 10 mL/kg.

-Deferoxamine (Desferal) 15 mg/kg/hr x 48 hours (max 12 gm/day) concomitantly with transfusion or 1-2 gm/day SQ over 8-24 hrs.

-Vitamin C 100 mg PO qd while receiving deferoxamine.

-Vitamin E PO qd while receiving deferoxamine.

    <1 year: 100 IU/day

    1-6 year: 200 IU/day

    >6 year: 400 IU/day

-Penicillin VK (Pen Vee K) (prophylaxis for pneumococcal infections): <3 years: 125 mg PO bid; >3 years: 250 mg PO bid [elixir: 125 mg/5 mL, 250 mg/5 mL; tabs: 125, 250, 500 mg]. If compliance with oral antibiotics is poor, use penicillin G benzathine 50,000 U/kg (max 1.2 million units) IM every 3 weeks. Erythromycin is used if penicillin allergic.

10. **Extras and X-rays:** CXR.
11. **Labs:** CBC, blood culture and sensitivity, reticulocyte count, type and cross, SMA 7, parvovirus titers, UA, urine culture and sensitivity.

Kawasaki's Syndrome

1. **Admit to:**
2. **Diagnosis:**
3. **Condition:**
4. **Vital signs:** Call MD if:
5. **Activity:** Bedrest.
6. **Nursing:** Temperature at q4-6h.
7. **Diet:**
8. **Special Medications:**

-Immunoglobulin (IVIG) 2 gm/kg/dose IV x 1 dose. Administer dose at 0.02 mL/kg/min over 30 min; if no adverse reaction, increase to 0.04 mL/kg/min over 30 min; if no adverse reaction, increase to 0.08 mL/kg/min for remainder of infusion. Defer measles vaccination for 11 months after receiving high-dose IVIG [inj: 50 mg/mL, 100 mg/mL].

-Aspirin 100 mg/kg/day PO or PR q6h until fever resolves, then 8-10 mg/kg/day PO/PR qd [supp: 60, 120, 125, 130, 195, 200, 300, 325, 600, 650 mg; tabs: 325, 500, 650 mg; tab, chew: 81 mg].

-Ambubag, epinephrine (0.1 mL/kg of 1:10,000), and diphenhydramine 1 mg/kg (max 50 mg) should be available for IV use if an anaphylactic reaction to immunoglobulin occurs.

9. **Extras and X-rays:** ECG, echocardiogram, chest X-ray. Rheumatology consult.

10. **Labs:** CBC with differential and platelet count. ESR, CBC, liver function tests, rheumatoid factor, salicylate levels, blood culture and sensitivity x 2, SMA 7.

Fluids and Electrolytes

Dehydration

1. **Admit to:**
2. **Diagnosis:** Dehydration
3. **Condition:**
4. **Vital signs:** Call MD if:
5. **Activity:**
6. **Nursing:** Inputs and outputs, daily weights. Urine specific gravity q void.
7. **Diet:**
8. **IV Fluids:**

Maintenance Fluids:

<10 kg	100 mL/kg/24h
10-20 kg	1000 mL plus 50 mL/kg/24h for each kg >10 kg
>20 kg	1500 mL plus 20 mL/kg/24h for each kg >20 kg.

Electrolyte Requirements:

Sodium: 3-5 mEq/kg/day
Potassium: 2-3 mEq/kg/day
Chloride: 3 mEq/kg/day
Glucose: 5-10 gm/100 mL water required (D5W - D10W)

Estimation of Dehydration			
Degree of Dehydration	**Mild**	**Moderate**	**Severe**
Weight Loss - Infants	5%	10%	15%
Weight Loss - Children	3%-4%	6%-8%	10%
Pulse	Normal	Slightly increased	Very increased
Blood Pressure	Normal	Normal to orthostatic, >10 mm Hg change	Orthostatic to shock
Behavior	Normal	Irritable	Hyperirritable to lethargic
Thirst	Slight	Moderate	Intense
Mucous Membranes	Normal	Dry	Parched
Tears	Present	Decreased	Absent, sunken eyes

Degree of Dehydration	Mild	Moderate	Severe
Anterior Fontanelle	Normal	Normal to sunken	Sunken
External Jugular Vein	Visible when supine	Not visible except with supraclavicular pressure	Not visible even with supraclavicular pressure
Skin	Capillary refill <2 sec	Delayed capillary refill, 2-4 sec (decreased turgor)	Very delayed capillary refill (>4 sec), tenting; cool skin, acrocyanotic, or mottled
Urine Specific Gravity (SG)	>1.020	>1.020; oliguria	Oliguria or anuria
Approximate Fluid Deficit	<50 mL/kg	50-100 mL/kg	$\geq$100 mL/kg

Electrolyte Deficit Calculation:

Na^+ deficit = (desired Na - measured Na in mEq/L) x 0.6 x weight in kg

K^+ deficit = (desired K - measured K in mEq/L) x 0.25 x weight in kg

Cl^- deficit= (desired Cl - measured Cl in mEq/L) x 0.45 x weight in kg

Free H_2O deficit in hypernatremic dehydration = 4 mL/kg for every mEq that serum Na >145 mEq/L.

Phase 1, Acute Fluid Resuscitation (Symptomatic Dehydration):

-Give NS 20-30 mL/kg IV at maximum rate; repeat fluid boluses of NS 20-30 mL/kg until blood pressure and pulse are normal.

Phase 2, Deficit and Maintenance Therapy (Asymptomatic dehydration):

Hypotonic Dehydration (Na⁺ <125 mEq/L):

-Calculate total maintenance and deficit fluids and sodium deficit for 24h (minus fluids and electrolytes given in phase 1). If isotonic or hyponatremic dehydration, replace 50% over 8h and 50% over next 16h.

-Estimate and replace ongoing losses q6-8h.

-Add potassium to IV solution after first void.

-Usually D5 1/2 NS or D5 1/4 NS saline with 10-40 mEq KCL/liter 60 mL/kg over 2 hours. Then infuse at 6-8 mL/kg/h for 12h.

-See hyponatremia, page 111.

Isotonic Dehydration (Na⁺ 130-150 mEq/L):

-Calculate total maintenance and replacement fluids for 24h (minus fluids and electrolytes given in phase 1) and give half over first 8h, then remaining half over next 16 hours.

-Add potassium to IV solution after first void.

-Estimate and replace ongoing losses.

-Usually D5 1/2 NS or D5 1/4 NS with 10-40 mEq KCL/L.

Hypertonic Dehydration (Na⁺ >150 mEq/L):

- Calculate and correct free water deficit and correct slowly. Reduce serum sodium by 10 mEq/L/day; do not reduce sodium by more than 15 mEq/L/24h or by >0.5 mEq/L/hr.
- If volume depleted, give NS 20-40 mL/kg IV until adequate circulation, then give 1/2-1/4 NS in 5% dextrose to replace half of free water deficit over first 24h. Follow serial serum sodium levels and correct deficit over 48-72h.
- **Free water deficit:** 4 mL/kg x (serum Na⁺ -145)
- Also see "hypernatremia" page 111.
- Add potassium to IV solution after first void as KCL.
- Usually D5 1/4 NS or D5W with 10-40 mEq/L KCL. Estimate and replace ongoing losses and maintenance.

Replacement of ongoing losses (usual fluids):

- Nasogastric suction: D5 1/2 NS with 20 mEq KCL/L or 1/2 NS with KCL 20 mEq/L.
- Diarrhea: D5 1/4 NS with 40 mEq KCl/L

Oral Rehydration Therapy (mild-moderate dehydration <10%):

- Oral rehydration electrolyte solution (Rehydralyte, Pedialyte, Ricelyte, Revital Ice) deficit replacement of 60-80 mL/kg PO or via NG tube over 2h. Provide additional fluid requirement over remaining 18-20 hours; add anticipated fluid losses from stools of 10 mL/kg for each diarrheal stool.

Oral Electrolyte Solutions			
Product	**Na (mEq/L)**	**K (mEq/L)**	**Cl (mEq/L)**
Rehydralyte	75	20	65
Ricelyte	50	25	45
Pedialyte	45	20	35

Hyperkalemia

1. **Admit to:** Pediatric ICU.
2. **Diagnosis:** Hyperkalemia.
3. **Condition:**
4. **Vital signs:** Call MD if:
5. **Activity:**
6. **Nursing:** Continuous ECG monitoring, inputs and outputs, daily weights.
7. **Diet:**
8. **IV Fluids:**

Hyperkalemia (K⁺ >7 or EKG Changes)

-Calcium gluconate 50-100 mg/kg (max 1 gm) IV over 5-10 minutes or calcium chloride 10-20 mg/kg (max 1 gm) IV over 10 minutes.

-Regular insulin 0.1 U/kg plus glucose 0.5 gm/kg IV bolus (as 10% dextrose).

-Sodium bicarbonate 1-2 mEq/kg IV over 3-5 min (give after calcium in separate IV), repeat in 10-15 min if necessary.

-Furosemide (Lasix) 1 mg/kg/dose (max 40 mg IV) IV q6-12h prn, may increase to 2 mg/kg/dose IV [inj: 10 mg/mL].

-Kayexalate resin 0.5-1 gm/kg PO/PR. 1 gm resin binds 1 mEq of potassium.

9. **Extras and X-rays:** ECG, dietetics, consult.
10. **Labs:** SMA7, Mg, calcium, CBC, platelets. UA; urine potassium.

Hypokalemia

1. **Admit to:** Pediatric ICU
2. **Diagnosis:** Hypokalemia.
3. **Condition:**
4. **Vital signs:** Call MD if:
5. **Activity:**
6. **Nursing:** ECG monitoring, inputs and outputs, daily weights.
7. **Diet:**
8. **IV Fluids:**

If serum K >2.5 mEq/L and ECG changes are absent:

Add 20-40 mEq KCL/L to maintenance IV fluids. May give 1-4 mEq/kg/day to maintain normal serum potassium. May supplement with oral potassium.

K <2.5 mEq/L and ECG abnormalities:

Give KCL 1-2 mEq/kg IV at 0.5 mEq/kg/hr; max rate 1 mEq/kg/hr or 20 mEq/kg/hr in life-threatening situations (whichever is smaller). Recheck serum potassium, and repeat IV boluses prn; ECG monitoring required.

Oral Potassium Therapy:

-Potassium chloride (KCl) elixir 1-3 mEq/kg/day PO q8-24h [10% soln = 1.33 mEq/mL].

9. **Extras and X-rays:** ECG, dietetics, consult.
10. **Labs:** SMA7, Mg, calcium, CBC. UA, urine potassium.

Hypernatremia

1. **Admit to:**
2. **Diagnosis:** Hypernatremia.
3. **Condition:**
4. **Vital signs:** Call MD if:
5. **Activity:**
6. **Nursing:** Inputs and outputs; daily weights.
7. **Diet:**
8. **IV Fluids:**

   If volume depleted or hypotensive, give NS 20-40 mL/kg IV until blood pressure and pulse are normal, then give D5 1/2 NS IV to replace half of body water deficit over first 24h. Correct serum sodium slowly at 0.5-1 mEq/L/hr. Correct remaining deficit over next 48-72h.

   Body water deficit (liter) = 0.6 x (weight kg) x (serum Na -140)

Hypernatremia with ECF Volume Excess:

   -Furosemide (Lasix) 1 mg/kg IV.

   -D5 1/4 NS to correct body water deficit.

9. **Extras and X-rays:** ECG.
10. **Labs:** SMA 7, osmolality, triglycerides. UA, urine specific gravity; 24h urine Na, K, creatinine.

Hyponatremia

1. **Admit to:**
2. **Diagnosis:** Hyponatremia.
3. **Condition:**
4. **Vital signs:** Call MD if:
5. **Activity:**
6. **Nursing:** Inputs and outputs, daily weights, neurochecks.
7. **Diet:**
8. **IV Fluids:**

Hyponatremia with Edema (Hypervolemia) (low osmolality <280 urine sodium <10 mM/L: nephrosis, CHF, cirrhosis; urine sodium >20: acute/chronic renal failure):

   -Water restrict to half maintenance.

   -Furosemide (Lasix) 1 mg/kg/dose IV over 1-2 min or 2-3 mg/kg/day PO q8-24h.

Hyponatremia with Normal Volume Status (low osmolality <280, urine sodium <10 mM/L: water intoxication; urine sodium >20 mM/L: SIADH, hypothyroidism, renal failure, Addison's disease, stress, drugs):

   -0.9% saline with 20-40 mEq KCL/L infused to correct hyponatremia at rate of <0.5 mEq/L/hr **OR** use 3% saline in severe hyponatremia [3% saline = 513 mEq/liter].

Hyponatremia with Hypovolemia (low osmolality <280; urine sodium <10 mM/L: vomiting, diarrhea, 3rd space/respiratory/skin loss; urine sodium >20 mM/L: diuretics, renal injury, renal tubular acidosis, adrenal insufficiency, partial obstruction, salt wasting):

-If volume depleted, give NS 20-40 mL/kg IV until adequate circulation.

-Gradually correct sodium deficit in increments of 10 mEq/L. Determine volume deficit clinically, and determine sodium deficit as below.

-Calculate 24 hour fluid and sodium requirement and give half over first 8 hours, then give remainder over 16 hours. 0.9% saline = 154 mEq/L

-Usually D5NS 60 mL/kg IV over 2h (this will increase extracellular sodium by 10 mEq/L), then infuse at 6-8 mL/kg/hr x 12h.

Severe Symptomatic Hyponatremia:

-If volume depleted, give NS 20-40 mL/kg until adequate circulation.

-Determine volume of 3% hypertonic saline (513 mEq/L) to be infused as follows:

Na(mEq) deficit = 0.6 x (wt kg) x (desired Na - actual Na)

Volume of soln (L) = Sodium to be infused (mEq) ÷ mEq/L in solution

-Correct half of sodium deficit slowly over 24h.

-For acute correction, the serum sodium goal is 125 mEq/L; max rate for acute replacement is 1 mEq/kg/hr. Serum Na should be adjusted in increments of 5 mEq/L to reach 125 mEq/L. The first dose is given over 4 hrs. For further correction for serum sodium to above 125 mEq/L, calculate mEq dose of sodium and administer over 24-48h.

9. Extras and X-rays: CXR, ECG.

10. Labs: SMA 7, osmolality, triglyceride. UA, urine specific gravity. Urine osmolality, Na, K; 24h urine Na, K, creatinine.

Hypophosphatemia

Indications for Intermittent IV Administration:

1. Serum phosphate <1.0 mg/dL or
2. Serum phosphate <2.0 mg/dL and patient symptomatic or
3. Serum phosphate <2.5 mg/dL and patient on ventilator

Treatment of Hypophosphatemia		
Dosage of IV Phosphate		**Serum Phosphate**
Low dose	0.08 mM/kg IV over 6 hrs	>1 mg/dL
Intermediate dose	0.16 mM/kg IV over 6 hrs 0.24 mM/kg IV over 4 hrs	0.5-1 mg/dL
High Dose	0.36 mM/kg IV over 6 hrs	<0.5 mg/dL

IV Phosphate Cations:
  Sodium phosphate: Contains sodium 4 mEq/mL, phosphate 3 mM/mL
  Potassium phosphate: Contains potassium 4.4 mEq/mL, phosphate 3 mM/mL
  Max rate 0.06 mM/kg/hr

Oral Phosphate Replacement

1-3 mM/kg/day PO bid-qid

Potassium Phosphate:

  Powder (Neutra-Phos-K): phosphorus 250 mg [8 mM] and potassium 556 mg [14.25 mEq] per packet; Tab (K-Phos Original): phosphorus 114 mg [3.7 mM], potassium 144 mg [3.7 mEq]

Sodium Phosphate: Phosphosoda Soln per 100 mL: sodium phosphate 18 gm and sodium biphosphate 48 gm [contains phosphate 4 mM/mL]

Sodium and Potassium Phosphate: Powd Packet: phosphorus 250 mg [8 mM], potassium 278 mg [7.125 mEq], sodium 164 mg [7.125 mEq];
  Tabs:
  K-Phos MF: phosphorus 125.6 mg [4 mM], potassium 44.5 mg [1.1 mEq], sodium 67 mg [2.9 mEq]
  K-Phos Neutral: phosphorus 250 mg [8 mM], potassium 45 mg [1.1 mEq], sodium 298 mg [13 mEq]
  K-Phos No 2: phosphorus 250 mg [8 mM], potassium 88 mg [2.3 mEq], sodium 134 mg [5.8 mEq]
  Uro-KP-Neutral: phosphorus 250 mg [8 mM], potassium 49.4 mg [1.27 mEq], sodium 250.5 mg [10.9 mEq]

Hypomagnesemia

Indications for Intermittent IV Administration:
1. Serum magnesium <1.2 mg/dL.
2. Serum magnesium <1.6 mg/dL and patient symptomatic.
3. Calcium-resistant tetany.

Magnesium Sulfate, Acute Treatment:
-25-50 mg/kg/dose (0.2-0.4 mEq/kg/dose) IV every 4-6 hrs x 3-4 doses as needed (max 2000 mg = 16 mEq/dose); max rate 1 mEq/kg/hr (125 mg/kg/hr).

Magnesium Sulfate IV Maintenance Dose: 1-2 mEq/kg/day (125-250 mg/kg/day) in maintenance IV solution.

Magnesium PO Maintenance Dose: 10-20 mg/kg/dose **elemental magnesium** PO qid.

Magnesium Chloride (Slow-Mag): mg salt (mEq elemental magnesium; mg elemental magnesium)
Tab, SR: 535 mg (5.2 mEq; 63 mg).

Magnesium Gluconate (Magonate): mg salt (mEq elemental magnesium; mg elemental magnesium)
Liq: 1000 mg/5mL (4.8 mEq/5mL; 54 mg).
Tab: 500 mg (2.4 mEq; 27 mg).

Magnesium Oxide: mg salt (mEq elemental magnesium; mg elemental magnesium).
Tabs: 400 mg (20 mEq; 242 mg), 420 mg (21 mEq; 254 mg), 500 mg (25 mEq; 302 mg).
Caps: 140 mg (7 mEq; 84 mg).

Magnesium Sulfate: mg salt (mEq elemental magnesium; mg elemental magnesium)
Soln: 500 mg/mL (4.1 mEq/mL; 49.3 mg/mL).

Newborn Care

Neonatal Resuscitation

APGAR Score			
Sign	0	1	2
Heart rate per minute	Absent	Slow (<100)	>100
Respirations	Absent	Slow, irregular	Good, crying
Muscle tone	Limp	Some flexion	Active motion
Reflex irritability	No response	Grimace	Cough or sneeze
Color	Blue or pale	Pink body with blue extremities	Completely pink

Assess APGAR score at 1 minute and 5 minutes, then continue assessment at 5 minute intervals until APGAR is greater than 7.

General Measures:
1. Review history, check equipment, oxygen, masks, laryngoscope, ET tubes, medications.

Vigorous, Crying Infant: Provide routine delivery room care for infants with heart rate >100 beats per minute, spontaneous respirations, and good color and tone: provide warmth, clear the airway, and dry the infant.

Meconium in Amniotic Fluid:
1. Deliver the head and suction meconium from the hypopharynx on delivery of the head. If the newly born infant has absent or depressed respirations, heart rate <100 bpm, or poor muscle tone, perform direct tracheal suctioning to remove meconium from the airway.
2. If no improvement occurs or if the clinical condition deteriorates, bag and mask ventilate with intermittent positive pressure using 100% FiO_2; stimulate vigorously by drying. Initial breath pressure: 30-40 cm H_2O for term infants, 20-30 cm H_2O for preterm infants. Ventilate at 15-20 cm H_2O at 30-40 breaths per minute. Monitor bilateral breath sounds and

expansion.

3. If spontaneous respirations develop and heart rate is normal, gradually reduce ventilation rate until using only continuous positive airway pressure (CPAP) is required. Wean to blow-by oxygen, but continue blow-by oxygen if the baby remains dusky.

4. Consider intubation if the heart rate remains <100 beats per minute and is not rising, or if respirations are poor and weak.

Resuscitation:

1. Provide assisted ventilation if stimulation does not achieve prompt onset of spontaneous respirations or the heart rate is <100 bpm.

2. Provide chest compressions if the heart rate is absent or remains <60 bpm despite adequate assisted ventilation for 30 seconds. Coordinate chest compressions with ventilations at a ratio of 3:1 and a rate of 120 events per minute to achieve 90 compressions and 30 breaths per minute.

3. Chest compressions should be done by two thumb-encircling hands. The depth of chest compression should be one third of the anterior-posterior diameter of the chest. Chest compressions should be sufficiently deep to generate a palpable pulse.

4. If condition worsens or if there is no change after 30 seconds, or if mask ventilation is difficult: use laryngoscope to suction oropharynx and trachea and intubate. Apply positive pressure ventilation. Check bilateral breath sounds and chest expansion. Check and adjust ET tube position if necessary. Continue cardiac compressions if heart rate remains depressed. Check CXR for tube placement.

Hypotension or Bradycardia or Asystole: Epinephrine 0.1-0.3 mL/kg [0.01-0.03 mg/kg (0.1 mg/mL = 1:10,000)] IV or ET q3-5min. Dilute ET dose to 2-3 mL in NS. If infant fails to respond, consider increasing dose to 0.1 mg/kg (0.1 mL/kg of 1 mg/mL = 1:1000).

Hypovolemia: Insert umbilical vein catheter and give O negative blood, plasma, 5% albumin, Ringer's lactate, or normal saline 10 mL/kg IV over 5-10 minutes. Repeat as necessary to correct hypovolemia.

Severe Birth Asphyxia, Mixed Respiratory/Metabolic Acidosis (not responding to ventilatory support; pH <7.2): Give sodium Bicarbonate 1 mEq/kg; dilute 1:1 in sterile water IV q5-10min as indicated.

Narcotic-Related Depression:

1. Naloxone (Narcan) 0.1 mg/kg = 0.25 mL/kg (0.4 mg/mL concentration) or 0.1 mL/kg (1 mg/mL concentration) ET/IV/IM/SC, may repeat q2-3 min. May cause drug withdrawal and seizures in the infant if the mother is a drug abuser.

Endotracheal Tube Sizes			
Weight (gm)	Gestational Age (weeks)	Tube Size (mm)	Depth of Insertion from Upper Lip (cm)
<1000	<28	2.5	6.5-7
1000-2000	28-34	3	37079
2000-3000	34-38	3.5	37111
>3000	>38	3.5-4.0	>9

Suspected Neonatal Sepsis

1. **Admit to:**
2. **Diagnosis:** Suspected sepsis
3. **Condition:**
4. **Vital signs:** Call MD if:
5. **Activity:**
6. **Nursing:** Inputs and outputs, daily weights, tepid sponge baths prn temp >38°C, consent for lumbar puncture.
7. **Diet:**
8. **IV Fluids:** IV fluids at 1-1.5 times maintenance.
9. **Special Medications:**

Newborn Infants <1 month old (group B strep, E coli, or group D strep, gram negatives, Listeria monocytogenes):

-Ampicillin and gentamicin **OR** ampicillin and cefotaxime as below.

-Add vancomycin as below if >7 days old and a central line is present.

Neonatal Dosage of Ampicillin:

<1200 gm 0-4 weeks: 100 mg/kg/day IV/IMq12h

1200-2000 gm:

≤7d: 100 mg/kg/day IV/IM q12h

>7d: 150 mg/kg/day IV/IM q8h

>2000 gm:

≤7d: 150 mg/kg/day IV/IM q8h

>7d: 200 mg/kg/day IV/IM q6h

Cefotaxime (Claforan):
   <1200 grams: 0-4 wks: 100 mg/kg/day IV/IM q12h
   $\geq$1200 grams: 0-7 days: 100 mg/kg/day IV/IM q12h
      >7 days: 150 mg/kg/day IV/IM q8h
Gentamicin (Garamycin)/tobramycin (Nebcin):
   <1200 gm 0-4 weeks: 2.5 mg/kg/dose IV/IMq24h
   1200-2000 gm:
      $\leq$7d: 2.5 mg/kg/dose IV/IM q12-24h
      >7d: 2.5 mg/kg/dose IV/IM q12-24h
   >2000 gm:
      $\leq$7d: 2.5 mg/kg/dose IV/IM q12-24h
      >7d: 2.5 mg/kg/dose IV/IM q12h
Neonatal Vancomycin (Vancocin) Dosage:
   <1200 gm 0-4 weeks: 15 mg/kg/dose IV q24h
   1200-2000 gm:
      $\leq$7d: 10 mg/kg/dose IV q12-18h
      >7d: 10 mg/kg/dose IV q8-12h
   >2000 gm:
      $\leq$7d: 10 mg/kg/dose IV q12h
      >7d: 10 mg/kg/dose IV q8-12h
Nafcillin (Nafcil):
   <1200 gm:
      0-4 weeks 50 mg/kg/day IV/IM q12h
   1200-2000 gm:
      $\leq$7 days: 50 mg/kg/day IV/IM q12h
      >7 days: 75 mg/kg/day IV/IM q8h
   >2000 gm:
      $\leq$7 days: 75 mg/kg/day IV/IM q8h
      >7 days: 100 mg/kg/day IV/IM q6h
Mezlocillin (Mezlin):
   <1200 gm:
      0-4 weeks 150 mg/kg/day IV/IM q12h
   1200-2000 gm:
      $\leq$7 days: 150 mg/kg/day IV/IM q12h
      >7 days: 225 mg/kg/day IV/IM q8h
   >2000 gm:
      $\leq$7 days: 150 mg/kg/day IV/IM q12h
      >7 days: 225 mg/kg/day IV/IM q8h
Amikacin:
   <1200 gm 0-4 weeks: 10 mg/kg/dose IV/IM q24h
   1200-2000 gm:
      $\leq$7d: 10 mg/kg/dose IV/IM q12-24h
      >7d: 10 mg/kg/dose IV/IM q12-24h

>2000 gm:
$\leq$7d: 10 mg/kg/dose IV/IM q12-24h
>7d: 10 mg/kg/dose IV/IM q12h
10. **Extras and X-rays:** CXR
10. **Laboratory Studies:** CBC, SMA 7, blood culture and sensitivity; UA, culture and sensitivity, antibiotic levels.

CSF Tube 1 - Gram stain, bacterial culture and sensitivity, antigen screen (1-2 mL).

CSF Tube 2 - Glucose protein (1-2 mL).

CSF Tube 3 - Cell count and differential (1-2 mL).

Respiratory Distress Syndrome

1. Provide mechanical ventilation as indicated.
2. Exogenous surfactant:

Prophylactic Therapy: Infants at risk for developing RDS with a birth weight <1250 gm.

Rescue Therapy: Treatment of infants with RDS based on respiratory distress not attributable to any other causes and chest radiographic findings consistent with RDS.

-Beractant (Survanta): 4 mL/kg of birth weight via endotracheal tube then q6h up to 4 doses total [100 mg (4 mL), 200 mg (8 mL)]

-Colfosceril (Exosurf): 5 mL/kg of birth weight via endotracheal tube then q12h for 2-3 doses total [108 mg (10 mL)]

-Poractant alfa (Curosurf): first dose 2.5 mL/kg (200 mg/kg/dose) of birthweight via endotracheal tube, may repeat with 1.25 mL/kg/dose (100 mg/kg/dose) at 12-hour intervals for up to two additional doses [120 mg (1.5 mL), 240 mg (3 mL)]

-Calfactant (Infasurf): 3 mL/kg via endotracheal tube, may repeat q12h up to a total of 3 doses [6 mL]

Necrotizing Enterocolitis

Treatment:
1. Decompress bowel with a large-bore (10 or 12 French), double-lumen nasogastric or orogastric tube, and apply intermittent suction.
2. Replace fluid losses with IV fluids; monitor urine output, tissue perfusion and blood pressure; consider central line monitoring.
3. Give blood and blood products for anemia, thrombocytopenia, or coagulopathy. Monitor abdominal X-rays for free air from perforation.

4. **Antibiotics:** Ampicillin and gentamicin or tobramycin or cefotaxime. Add vancomycin if a central line is present.
5. **Diagnostic evaluation:** Serial abdominal X-rays with lateral decubitus, CBC with differential and platelets; DIC panel, blood cultures x 2; Wright's stain of stool; stool cultures.
6. Monitor the patient frequently for perforation, electrolyte disturbances, and radiologic evidence of pneumatosis intestinalis and portal vein gas. Obtain surgical evaluation if perforation is suspected.

Apnea

1. **Admit to:**
2. **Diagnosis:** Apnea.
3. **Condition:**
4. **Vital signs:** Call MD if:
5. **Activity:**
6. **Nursing:** Heart rate monitor, impedance apnea monitor, pulse oximeter. Keep bag and mask resuscitation equipment at bed side. Rocker bed or oscillating water bed.
7. **Diet:** Infant formula ad lib
8. **IV Fluids:**
9. **Special Medications:**

Apnea of Prematurity/Central Apnea:
   -Aminophylline: loading dose 5 mg/kg IV, then maintenance 5 mg/kg/day IV q12h [inj: 25 mg/mL] **OR**
   -Theophylline: loading dose 5 mg/kg PO, then 5 mg/kg/day PO q12h. [elixir: 80 mg/15mL].
   -Caffeine citrate: Loading dose 10-20 mg/kg IV/PO, then 5 mg/kg/day PO/IV q12-24h [inj: 20 mg/mL, oral soln: 20 mg/mL. Oral suspension: 10 mg/mL].
10. **Extras and X-rays:** Pneumogram, cranial ultrasound. Upper GI (rule out reflux), EEG.
11. **Labs:** CBC, SMA 7, glucose, calcium, theophylline level (therapeutic range 6-14 mcg/mL) , caffeine level (therapeutic range 10-20 mcg/mL).

Chronic Lung Disease (Respiratory Distress Syndrome)

1. **Admit to:**
2. **Diagnosis:** Chronic lung disease.
3. **Condition:**

4. **Vital signs:** Call MD if:
5. **Activity:**
6. **Nursing:** Inputs and outputs, daily weights
7. **Diet:**
8. **IV Fluids:** Isotonic fluids at maintenance rate.
9. **Special Medications:**

Diuretics:

-Furosemide (Lasix) 1 mg/kg/dose PO/IV/IM q6-24h prn [inj: 10 mg/mL; oral soln: 10 mg/mL, 40 mg/5mL].

-Chlorothiazide (Diuril) 2-8 mg/kg/day IV q12-24h or 20-40 mg/kg/day PO q12h [inj: 500 mg; susp: 250 mg/5mL] **OR**

-Spironolactone (Aldactone) 2-3 mg/kg/day PO q12-24h [tabs: 25, 50, 100 mg; suspension].

Steroids:

-Dexamethasone (Decadron) 0.5-1 mg/kg/day IV/IM q6-12h **OR**

-Prednisone 1-2 mg/kg/day PO q12-24h [soln: 1 mg/mL, 5 mg/mL].

10. **Extras and X-rays:** CXR.
11. **Labs:** CBC, SMA 7.

Hyperbilirubinemia

1. **Admit to:**
2. **Diagnosis:** Hyperbilirubinemia.
3. **Condition:** Guarded.
4. **Vital signs:** Call MD if
5. **Activity:**
6. **Nursing:** Inputs and outputs, daily weights, monitor skin color, monitor for lethargy and hypotonia.
7. **Diet:**
8. **IV Fluids:** Isotonic fluids at maintenance rate (100-150 mL/kg/day). Encourage enteral feedings if possible.
9. **Special Medications:**

-Phenobarbital 5 mg/kg/day PO/IV q12-24h [elixir: 15 mg/5mL, 20 mg/5mL; inj: 30 mg/mL, 60 mg/mL, 65 mg/mL, 130 mg/mL].

-Phototherapy if bilirubin level is above 15-20 mg/dL.

-Exchange transfusion for severely elevated bilirubin.

10. **Symptomatic Medications:**
11. **Extras and X-rays:**
12. **Labs:** Total bilirubin, indirect bilirubin, albumin, SMA 7. Blood group typing of mother and infant, a direct Coombs' test. Complete blood cell count, reticulocyte count, blood smear. In infants of Asian or Greek descent, glucose-6-phosphate dehydrogenase (G6PD) should be measured.

Congenital Syphilis

Treatment:
- Penicillin G aqueous: 50,000 U/kg/dose IV/IM; 0-7 days of age: q12h; >7 days: q8h. Treat for 10-14 days. If one or more days is missed, restart entire course **OR**
- Procaine penicillin G 50,000 U/kg/day IM qd for 10-14 day.
- Obtain follow-up serology at 3, 6, 12 months until nontreponemal test is non-reactive. Infectious skin precautions should be taken.

Congenital Herpes Simplex Infection

- Acyclovir (Zovirax) 60 mg/kg/day IV q8h. Infuse each dose over 1 hr x 14 days (if disease is limited to skin, eye, and mouth) or 21 days (if disease is disseminated or involves the CNS). Infants with ocular involvement should also receive topical ophthalmic trifluridine.
- Trifluridine ophthalmic solution (Viroptic) 1 drop in each affected eye q2h while awake [ophth soln 1%: 7.5 mL bottle].

Patent Ductus Arteriosus

Treatment:
1. Restrict fluids if the infant is symptomatic.
2. Provide respiratory support and maintain hematocrit at 40%.
3. Furosemide (Lasix) 1-2 mg/kg/dose q6-8h PO.
4. **Indomethacin (Indocin):**

Indomethacin – Three dose course:			
Age at First Dose	Dose 1 (mg/kg/dose)	Dose 2 (mg/kg/dose)	Dose 3 (mg/kg/dose)
<48h	0.2	0.1	0.1
2-7d	0.2	0.2	0.2

Age at First Dose	Dose 1 (mg/kg/dose)	Dose 2 (mg/kg/dose)	Dose 3 (mg/kg/dose)
>7d	0.2	0.25	0.25

Give q12-24h IV over 20-30 min. Check serum creatinine and urine output prior to each dose.

Indomethacin – Five-dose course: 0.1 mg/kg/dose IV q24h x 5 days. Check serum creatinine and urine output prior to each dose.

1. **Diagnostic Considerations:** ABG, chest X-ray, ECG, CBC, electrolytes. Echocardiogram (to determine if PDA has closed).
2. Consider surgical intervention if two courses of indomethacin fail to close the PDA or if indomethacin therapy is contraindicated (hemodynamically unstable, renal impairment).

Hepatitis Prophylaxis

Infant born to HBs-Ag Positive Mother or Unknown Status Mother:
-Hepatitis B immune globulin (HBIG) 0.5 mL IM x 1 within 12 hours of birth
AND
-Hepatitis B vaccine 0.5 mL IM (at separate site) within 12 hours of birth, second dose at age 1-2 months, third dose at age 6 months.

Neonatal HIV Prophylaxis

1. Pregnant women with HIV should be given oral zidovudine (200 mg PO q8h or 300 mg PO q12h) beginning at 14 weeks gestation and continuing throughout the pregnancy.
2. Intravenous zidovudine should be given to the mother during labor until delivery (2 mg/kg during the first hour and then 1 mg/kg/hr until delivery).
3. Oral administration of zidovudine to the newborn should be instituted immediately after birth and continued for at least six weeks (start at 8mg/kg/day PO q6h for the first two weeks, and then follow the dosing regimens on page 57. The mother should not breast feed the infant.

Commonly Used Formulas

Normal urine output = 50 mL/kg/day
Oliguria <1 mL/kg/hr
Normal feedings = 5 ounces/kg/day
Formula = 20 kcal/ounce, 24 kcal/ounce, 27 kcal/ounce
Ounce = 30 mL
Caloric Needs = 100 kcal/kg/day
Calories/kg = mL of formula x 30 mL/ounce x kcal/ounce divided by weight.

Weight in kg = pounds divided by 2.2

Blood volume (mL) = 80 mL/kg x weight (kg)

Blood Products:
  10 mL/kg of PRBC will raise hematocrit 5%
  0.1 unit/kg platelets will raise platelet count by 25,000/mm^3
  1 U/kg of factor VIII will raise level by 2%

Cardiac output = HR x stroke volume

$$CO \text{ L/min} = \frac{125 \text{ mL O2/min/m}^2}{8.5 \{(1.36)(Hgb)(SaO2)\ (1.36)(Hgb)(SvO2)\}} \times 100$$

Anion Gap = Na - (Cl + HCO3)

$$Creatinine\ clearance = \frac{U\ Creatinine\ (mg/100\ mL)\ x\ U\ vol\ (mL)}{P\ Creatinine\ (mg/100\ mL)\ x\ time\ (1440\ min\ for\ 24h)}$$

$$Body\ water\ deficit\ (L) = \frac{0.6(weight\ kg)([Na\ serum]-140)}{140}$$

$$Osmolality = 2[Na + K] + \frac{BUN}{2.8} + \frac{glucose}{18} = NL\ 270\text{-}290\ mOsm/kg$$

$$Fractional\ excreted\ Na = \frac{U\ Na/\ Serum\ Na\ x\ 100}{U\ Creatinine/\ Serum\ Creatinine} = NL<1\%$$

$$Corrected\ serum\ Na+ = \frac{measured\ Na + serum\ glucose\ (mg/dL)}{36} = NL\ 140\ mEq/L$$

Basal energy expenditure (BEE):
  Males = 66 + (13.7 x actual weight in kg) + (5 x height in cm) - (6.8 x age)
  Females = 655 + (9.6 x actual weight in kg) + (1.7 x height in cm) - (4.7 x age)

Nitrogen Balance = Gm protein intake/6.25 - urine urea nitrogen - (3-4 gm/day insensible loss)

Normal Heart Rates		
Age	Range	Normal Rate (beats/min)
Newborn to 30 months	85-200	140
30 months to 2 years	100-190	130
2 years to 10 years	60-190	80
>10 years	50-100	75

Index

Order Form

Current Clinical Strategies books can also be purchased at all medical bookstores

Title	Book	CD
Treatment Guidelines in Medicine, 2006 Edition	$19.95	$36.95
Psychiatry History Taking, Third Edition	$12.95	$28.95
Psychiatry, 2006 Edition	$12.95	$28.95
Pediatric Drug Reference, 2004 Edition	$9.95	$28.95
Anesthesiology, 2004-2005 Edition	$16.95	$28.95
Medicine, 2005 Edition	$16.95	$28.95
Pediatric Treatment Guidelines, 2007 Edition	$19.95	$29.95
Physician's Drug Manual, 2005 Edition	$9.95	$28.95
Surgery, Sixth Edition	$12.95	$28.95
Gynecology and Obstetrics, 2006 Edition	$16.95	$30.95
Pediatrics, 2007 Edition	$12.95	$28.95
Family Medicine, 2006 Edition	$26.95	$46.95
History and Physical Examination in Medicine, Tenth Edition	$14.95	$28.95
Outpatient and Primary Care Medicine, 2005 Edition	$16.95	$28.95
Critical Care Medicine, 2007 Edition	$16.95	$32.95
Handbook of Psychiatric Drugs, 2005 Edition	$12.95	$28.95
Pediatric History and Physical Examination, Fourth Edition	$12.95	$28.95
Current Clinical Strategies CD-ROM Collection for Palm, Pocket PC, Windows, and Macintosh		$49.95

CD-ROMs are compatible with Palm, Pocket PC, Windows and Macintosh.

Quantity	Title	Amount

Order by Phone: 800-331-8227 or 949-348-8404
Fax: 800-965-9420 or 949-348-8405
Internet Orders: http://www.ccspublishing.com/ccs
Mail Orders:
Current Clinical Strategies Publishing
27071 Cabot Road, Suite 126
Laguna Hills, California 92653

Credit Card Number: _____

Exp: ____/____

A shipping charge of $5.00 will be added to each order

Signature: _____

Check Enclosed _____

Phone Number: (_____)_____

Name and Address (please print):

_____

_____

_____

_____